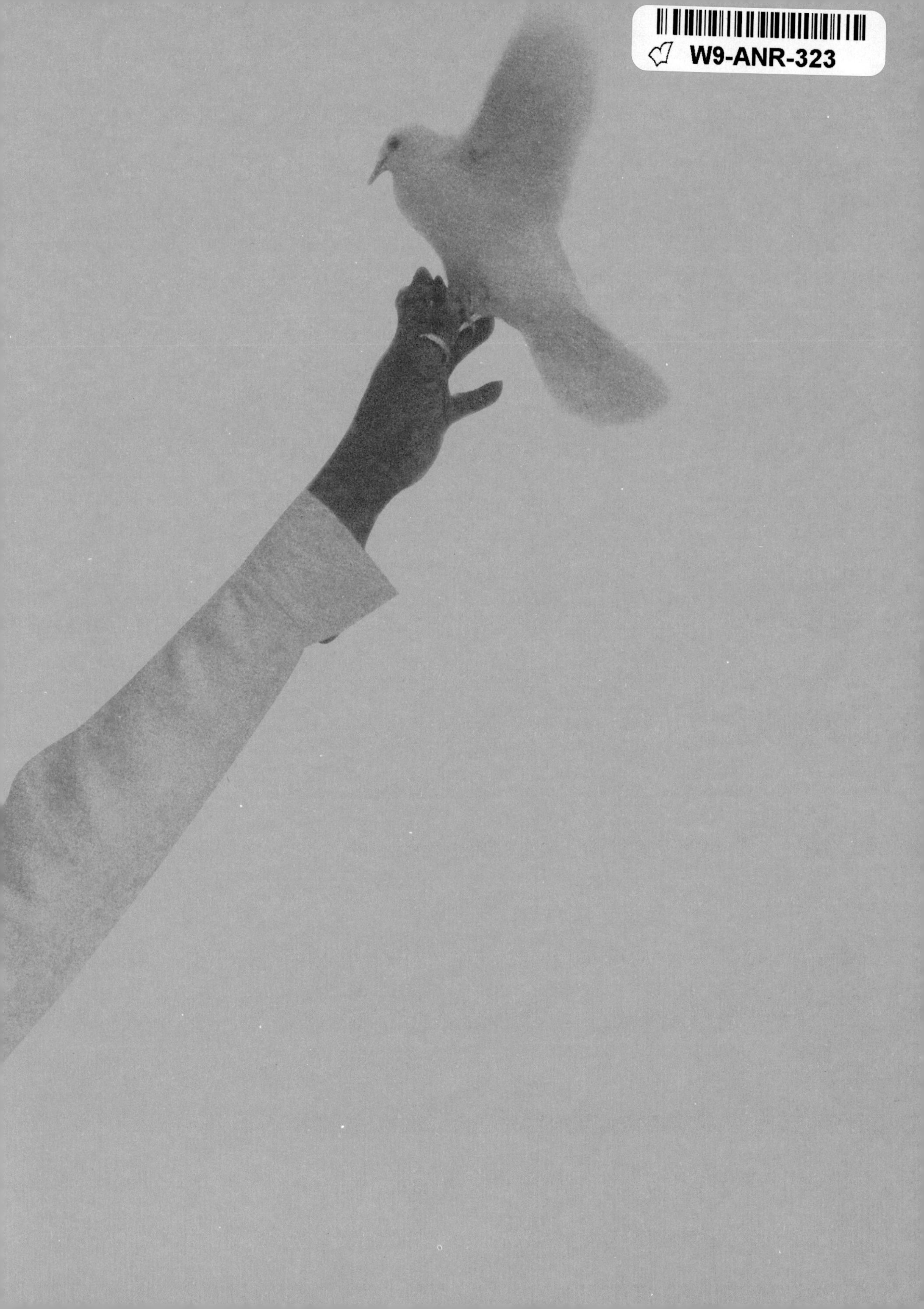

A New Plan for Success and Well-Being
from Today's Most Celebrated Women

women to WOMEN

Christina Lessa invites you to visit her website at
www.gobodymindsoul.com

First published in the United States of America in 2000
by UNIVERSE PUBLISHING
A Division of Rizzoli International Publications, Inc.
300 Park Avenue South
New York, NY 10010

Produced by CD Productions, New York, NY

2000 2001 2002 2003 2004 2005 / 10 9 8 7 6 5 4 3 2 1

Designed by Dan Petrucelli
Associate designer Heidi Volpe

Printed in Singapore

Library of Congress Cataloging-in-Publication Data

Lessa, Christina.
Women to women : a new plan for success and well being from today's most celebrated women / photography and interviews by Christina Lessa.
p. cm.
ISBN 0-7893-0356-6
1. Women--Life skills guides. 2. Women--Health and hygiene. 3. Women in the professions--Attitudes. I. Title.
HQ1221 .L637 2000
646.7'0082--dc21

00-055943

A New Plan for Success and Well-Being from Today's Most Celebrated Women

women to WOMEN

PHOTOGRAPHY AND INTERVIEWS BY
CHRISTINA LESSA

UNIVERSE

CONTENTS

INTROD

THE SKILL OF
SURVIVING ADVERSITY–
AND ACTUALLY GROWING IN
WISDOM AND STRENGTH
BECAUSE OF IT–
IS A SKILL ALL
WOMEN CAN DEVELOP.

UCTION

by Christina Lessa

There I was, **standing in front of the mirror in my bra and stockings,** hot rollers in my hair. As I breast-fed my two-week-old son with one hand, I applied mascara with the other like an old pro—all the while searching the ground for my shoe with my foot. I was getting ready for my first business meeting since giving birth to my only child. It was one of those moments when you see yourself from outside of your body and become aware of the reality of life in a new way. This is it, I thought. This is real life, maybe not life the way it was intended to be in the beginning, but life for a woman in the new millennium. All of a sudden I felt bonded to other women in a different way.

I was the youngest (by up to eighteen years) of seven children—the youthful one who had different ideas from anyone else's. I had always believed that my generational placement afforded me the luxury of being who I wanted to be. But the truth was talking back to me as I looked in the mirror that day. I wasn't unique from my sisters. I was exactly who they had groomed me to become by example.

My mind raced with memories of sitting on flowered bedspreads while they exposed me to some new facet of life. Sometimes it was as simple as watching them get ready for a date and marveling at the whole ritual, from careful clothing selection to makeup application. Other times it was more intense, like the time we waited on the bed anxiously as my sister Francesca told my father that she was dropping out of nursing school to open a flower shop at the age of nineteen. At times it was legendary, like the time my eldest and most obedient sister, Lucy, defied my mother by trading in her ribboned ponytails for a black armband in protest of Vietnam. There were sadder times as my parents split up and we all

body

huddled together as the fighting came to a head, debating who should go down this time and what tactic we could employ to try to help. A lot of the time fear would immobilize us and a secret call to the police would be our last resort. Every moment brought with it a new life lesson for my sisters and me.

Between the five of us we've shared the experiences of several generations. We've Elvised, Beatled, hippied, discoed, and punked. We've dated, married, divorced, remarried, miscarried, and had children. We have gone to college, graduate school, dropped out of high school, owned businesses, gone bankrupt, written books, become professors, secretaries, opera singers, waitresses, designers, and artists. We've been skinny and fat, Weight Watchered, aerobicized, and Stair Mastered, had numerous hair colors, and lived through decades of fads. We've worshiped, prayed, switched religions, left religion, and returned with a passion. Through all of this we have run the gamut of emotions together and have each grown closer to our potential as human beings. I was fortunate to have witnessed so much of this as a spectator, and I tried to pick up the right and the wrong of it all like a sponge. What burdens my sisters carried on their young shoulders as they ventured out into the world, especially in times that were much less kind to women. They were my mentors.

mind

As we all grew older we began to look to other women for advice and in turn shared it with one another. I still look forward to the times when we are all together to find out who got what where, and how they managed to accomplish this or that. It's an ongoing process and something I believe that all women do with each other. Throughout history women have passed down tips from one generation to the next—recipes, child-rearing advice, remedies for health problems. These hand-me-downs helped women survive generations of being denied formal education and other basic rights.

The networking of advice is what this book is all about. It's about women from strikingly different backgrounds who have achieved success in whatever area their passions led them, and the advice that they want to pass on. Many of them have overcome hardship and are living proof of the strength of the human spirit and the power of the mind. These women demonstrate what can happen when we strive for a quality life with purpose, and the information they offer us is the fruit of their labor.

In today's society women are expected to play so many different roles. We are often too busy to stop and wonder about the how and the why in the way we are living. The

WE ARE OFTEN TOO BUSY
TO STOP AND WONDER ABOUT THE HOW
AND THE WHY IN THE WAY WE ARE LIVING.
THE WOMEN IN THIS BOOK OFFER US INSIGHT
AND INSPIRATION FOR A BETTER LIFE.

women in this book offer us insight and inspiration for a better life. Their gifts of counsel cover many different topics within the body, mind, and soul. As we look to nurture our souls, spiritual advisor Iyanla Vanzant aids us by offering the benefits of self-introspection: "Self-celebration and affirmation are so lacking in women's lives today. They move from one thing to the next without really experiencing what they are doing. We need to begin to truly experience life, to isolate and identify what's driving us at any given time; only then do we have the opportunity to make a better choice." The skill of surviving adversity–and actually growing in wisdom and strength because of it–is one all women can develop. Drew Barrymore reflects on her victory over addiction and the lessons she's learned: "Women shouldn't be burdened by what existed in their past. We should all learn how to turn pain into strength."

When our minds are clear and receptive, a range of ideas can flow through them. The ideas offered by Dr. Christiane Northrup about health and the mind/body connection are the beginning of a new and improved thought process: "There is no illness that isn't emotional and mental as well as physical. When women change the basic conditions of their lives they heal faster, more completely, and with fewer medical interventions. Financial specialist Ellen McGirt and CEO Kim Polese urge women to continue to ask questions, consult experts, and not be afraid of something they don't know. Women can use their strengths in communication and building relationships to thrive in businesses that were formerly run only by men.

The body section brings with it a host of ideas for self-improvement. Fitness guru Kathy Smith reminds us that exercise is as much about improving the body as it is about boosting one's confidence: "Stop obsessing about whether or not your body is perfect. Just get out there and do something that makes you feel great." Bobbi Brown reinforces the enduring principle of feeling good through looking your best, with makeover ideas demonstrated on her six good friends, ranging in age from twenty to seventy.

soul

As I spent time with all of these women, one idea continued to resurface: that we must all strive to overcome the worry, stress, and overexertion that so many women face today and reconnect to our physical and spiritual selves without unnecessary self-criticism. We all agreed that in order to do this, we first have to determine the deeper meaning of our lives. We must abandon the idea that we are too busy for self-discovery as we open our eyes to the infinite possibilities of the world around us.

SO

The definition of soul seems very confused nowadays. We live in an age when people are not sure who or what they are, or whether or not their lives have any significant meaning. Do we really grow from rushing through life at the speed of light, being superwomen to everyone around us but forgetting our own souls? Does our spirit really become alive by changing spouses and jobs on impulse, undergoing plastic surgery, spending countless hours in therapy, or indulging in empty self-reflection over and over again? As I learned from Sister Mary Catherine in grade school, there is a world of difference between "you revolving around something" and "everything revolving around you."

Everyone longs for a life of significance. We all want to be thought of as having made a contribution to this world. Most of us have a deep desire to be validated and remembered for our accomplishments, both during and after our time on earth. In order to appreciate our own self-worth–and the value of those with whom we share our lives–we must develop a greater awareness of the world around us and our place in it. Iyanla Vanzant tells us to observe ourselves at all times; if we are making choices based on fear, guilt, or anger, she tells us to make another choice. I believe that in order to get real mileage out of self-reflection we must fully explore our spirituality and submit to a higher power.

The ability to pray was a gift my siblings and I were given as children. But there weren't any direct conversa-

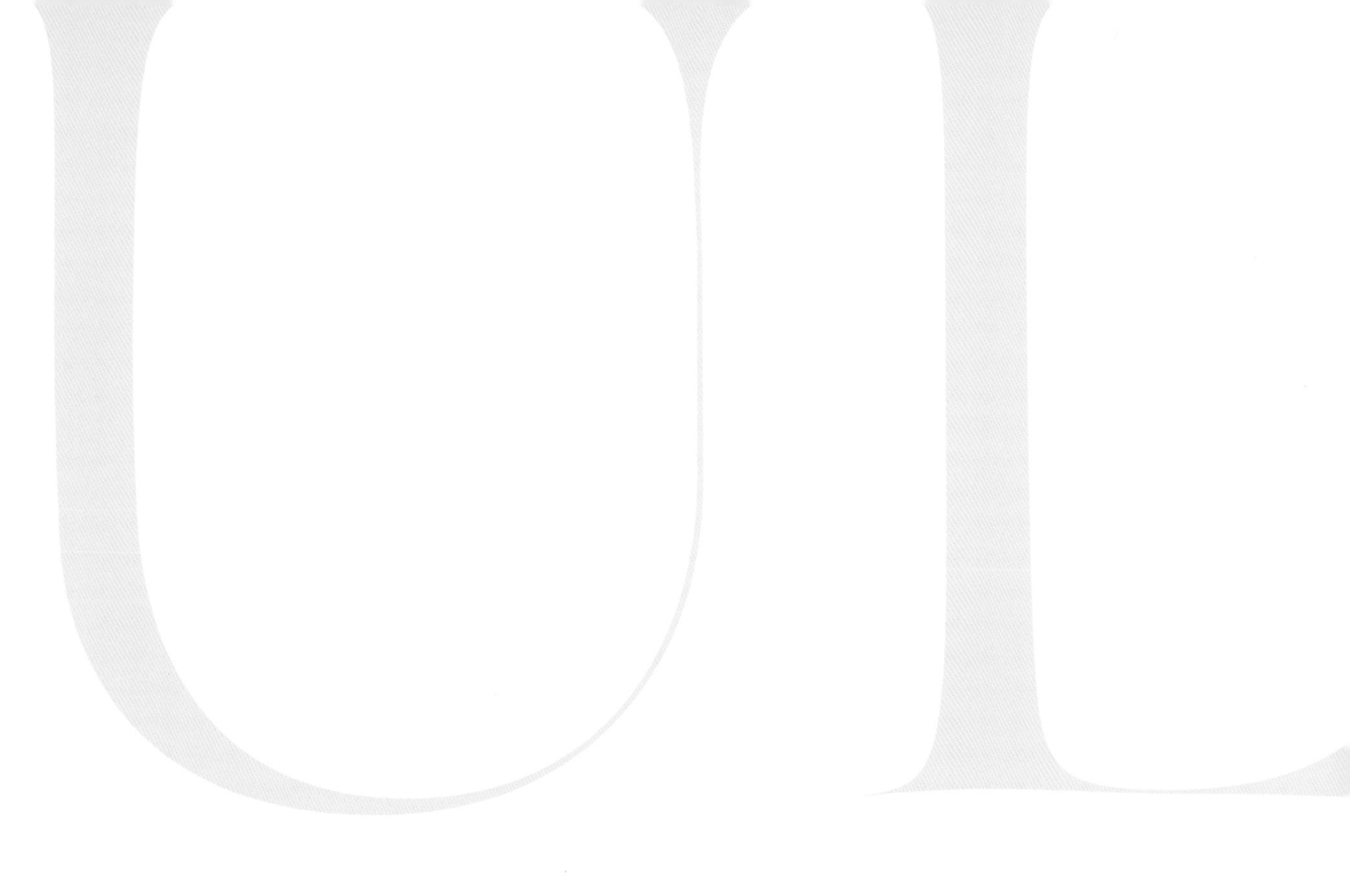

tions with God. When we would lose a shoe or a toy, my mother would tell us to pray to Saint Anthony. When my brother, a fireman, would rush off to sirens we called on Saint Christopher to protect him. If our cause had urgency there was always the Virgin Mary, and when all else failed, Saint Jude, the patron saint of lost causes, came to the rescue. Somehow it seemed taboo to go directly to the source. Now I can't imagine a day without talking to God. I always feel a little strange in the beginning, because there is this feeling that God already knows what you're about to say. It's the pure silence and simplicity of the prayer itself that brings out the true meaning in your unspoken words. When I listen carefully the answers usually lie in the questions that I ask.

Sarah Ban Breathnach reminds us that "loving ourselves into wholeness is not a frivolous luxury, it's the essence of our souls." This concept of spiritual beauty, when our inner growth is reflected in our outer packaging, is particularly poignant for women. It makes me think of my mother's bathrobe. Although it was old and covered with stains from a thousand breakfasts, she wore it religiously. Things being what they were, with seven children and a modest income, she rarely bought anything for herself, and certainly nothing of quality. But its frayed satin piping, numerous holes, and the giant safety pin that adorned her neckline became the nemesis of my Uncle John, who adored my mother. It was New Year's Day when Uncle John arrived carrying an enormous gift box. Everyone ran out to greet him, my mother in the robe. He presented the box to her and she opened it; inside was a very luxurious pink silk peignoir set. She resisted, he persisted, and before we knew it, he was helping her into her new robe. He held the ratty old one inches away from his lighter, and we watched as it went up in flames right on our front lawn. That night she put the new set neatly back in its box and, sadly, we never saw it on her again. It stayed in the box forever. She just couldn't own the pure luxury of it. It was a contradiction to her martyred lifestyle. When she shut that box she closed off a part of herself.

Too many women have boxed away a part of themselves out of fear—fear of nurturing their own souls. Here instead, are five women who live soulfully and beautifully in their own lives, each offering new ideas to help guide us through the journey of our spiritual paths.

IYANLA VANZANT

Spiritual life counselor Iyanla Vanzant is the award-winning and bestselling author of *Acts of Faith, In the Meantime, Yesterday I Cried,* and *One Day My Soul Just Opened Up.* As an empowerment specialist, spiritual counselor, and ordained minister, she lectures and facilitates workshops nationally with a mission to assist in the quest for spiritual enlightenment.

Q In your book *Yesterday I Cried* you describe overcoming tremendous obstacles to become an attorney, only to receive a higher calling just months into your first practice.

My purpose became clear and things just fell into place. I experienced the need for self-celebration and affirmation, which are so lacking in women's lives. They just go from one thing to the next without stopping to really experience what they are doing. They move from being a worker, to being a wife, to being a mother, to being a mother and a worker, and there is no place in between to just stop and reflect. We need to start to celebrate ourselves, honor our learning, and embrace ourselves fully along the way. If you don't take time to stop, grieve, feel, acknowledge–whatever it may be–that experience and the feelings and learning that come with it become worthless.

Q In *One Day My Soul Just Opened Up*, you tell us that we need to identify the specific emotion that is affecting us at a particular time, whether it's loneliness, discipline, guilt, or something else. That really struck me as a particularly appropriate insight for all women.

Life is about a total experience, but what we really want to do is become aware of what experience is impacting us at a particular time. If you don't understand that then you will find yourself doing and going and being in ways that are not supportive of you. For example, a woman who experiences a lot of guilt will always be trying to make up for the thing she feels guilty about. She may be overassuming responsibility for other people or things, always trying to clear up that guilt. She needs to take a breath and say, "What am I doing here? What am I feeling here? Why am I doing this? Why am I resentful about having to do this?" As we begin to isolate and identify what's driving us at any given time, then we have the opportunity to make a better choïce.

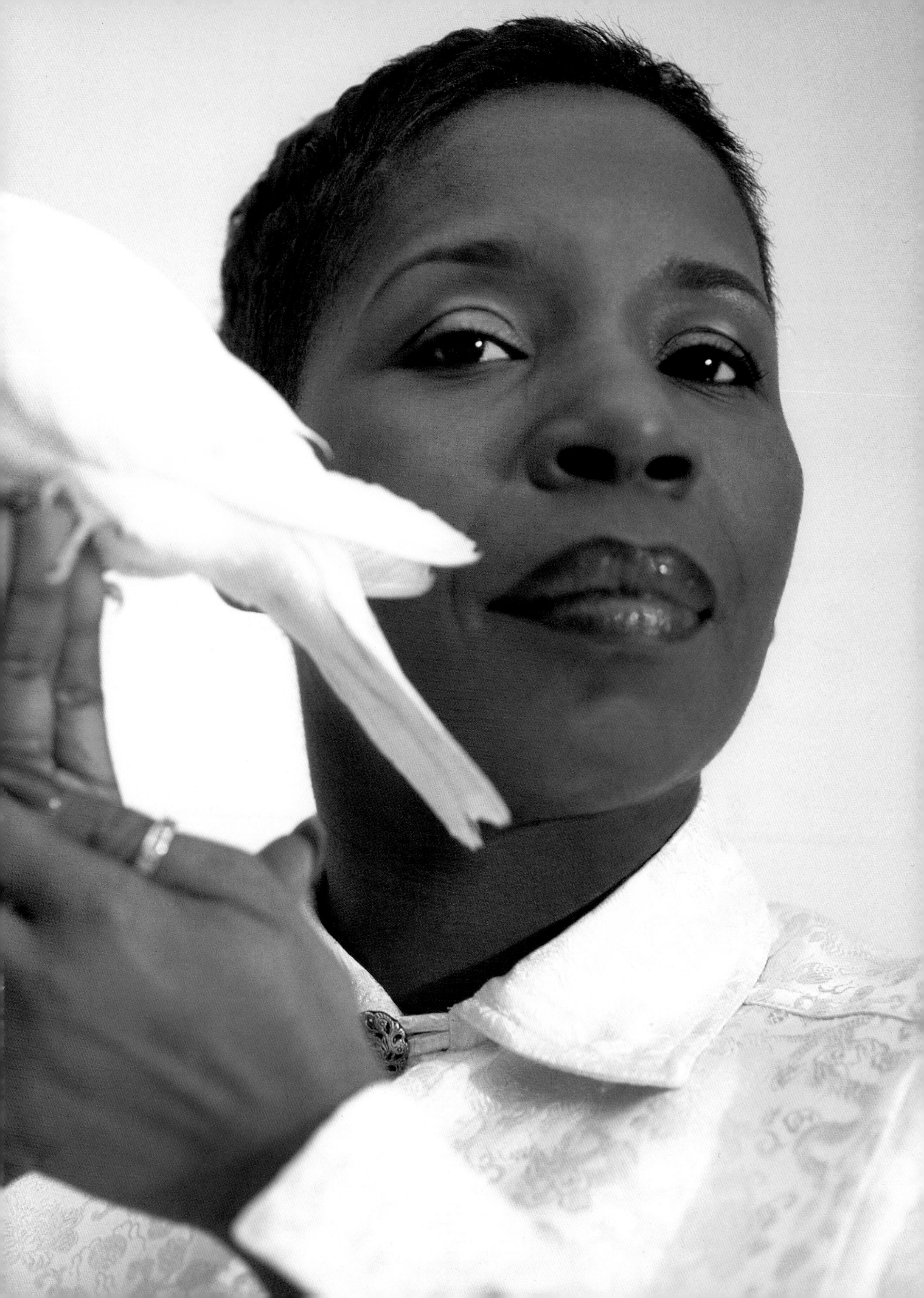

FEMININE
POWER IS SILENT,
DARK,
MYSTERIOUS,
HEALING,
NURTURING.

A WOMAN CAN WALK
INTO A ROOM
AND CONTROL IT.
SHE DOESN'T EVEN HAVE
TO OPEN HER MOUTH
IF SHE KNOWS
WHERE HER
POWER IS.

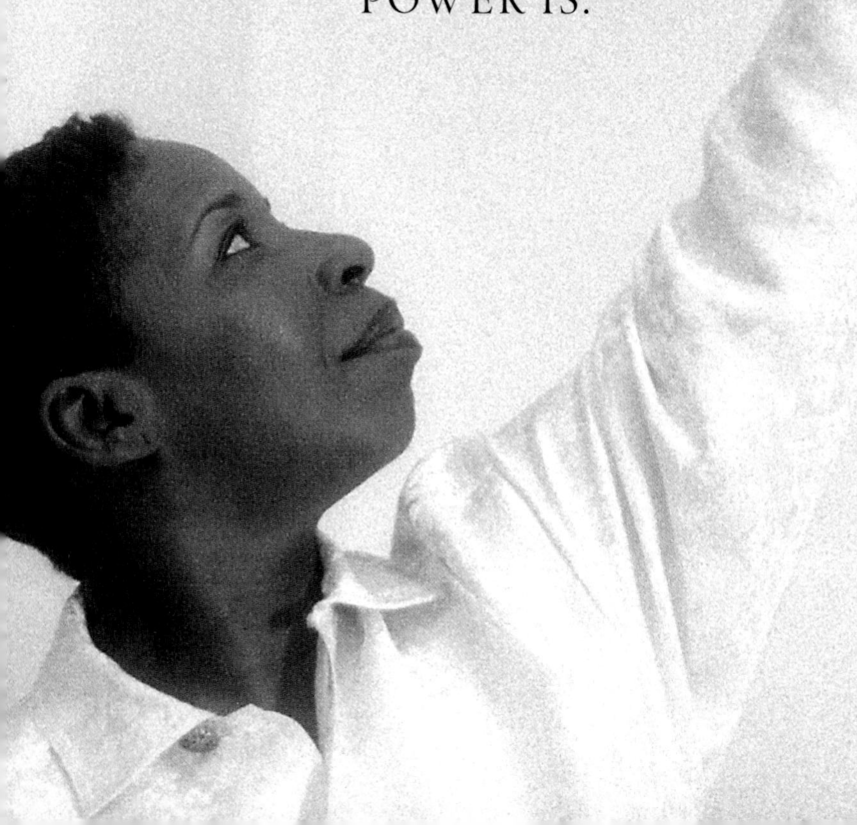

I often ask, are we driven or are we drawn? Are we driven to do certain things now to compensate for our experiences of the past? Or are we drawn to do certain things just based on our love and our open heart and our desire? I think that that's a question women should ask themselves at every opportunity. Am I driven to do this because of my unresolved past or am I drawn because of a deeper desire within me?

Q You went through so many things in life before your inspiration came. Everyone kept saying, "You'll see. You don't understand now, but just wait." I think being patient and trusting that answers will come is a rare and undervalued thing. We want it all now.

What does waiting mean? That's what we need to define first because some of us think that waiting is sitting there twiddling your thumbs and picking your nose until something befalls you. We think that today or tomorrow we're going to have this flash of inspiration that's going to save us from our dissatisfaction. But waiting is an ever-unfolding process. Someone doesn't just hand you understanding and clarity in an instant.

Life is all about waiting; each day is a kind of waiting–moving from one understanding to the next, from one revelation to the next, until you have that ultimate "Ah ha!" experience that allows you to put into practical application everything that's been revealed to you. That's waiting. It's not about sitting there waiting and doing nothing. It's not about "I'll do it when I lose five pounds or when I finish this book or when I master yoga or when the kids go to high school." Waiting is using the power of reflection and knowledge you gain to grow and move toward your passion and power.

Q Women today seem more empowered than ever—they're climbing the ladders at work without hitting the glass ceiling. Yet they seem to be giving their power away.

We don't even know what our power is! The question I used to ask women all the time is, "What is a feminine model of power?" But most women haven't seen one, so they keep doing things the way guys do them–being competitive and controlling, practicing one-upmanship. Those are not feminine forms of power. Feminine power is silent, dark, mysterious, healing, nurturing. A woman can walk into a room and control it. She doesn't even have to open her mouth if she knows where her power is.

Q The lack of feminine power is especially important now that computers, the internet, and technology—which are all very male-dominated fields—are redefining our world.

Nature is so wonderful, and yet we are continuing to move away from it. If we just watched nature, we would understand how to live. How long does it take for a tree to shed its leaves? And then how long does it take for those leaves to grow back? If we know this, we are learning that the shedding and the growing takes time. How long does it take for an egg to become an embryo, and an embryo to become a fetus, and a fetus to become a baby? Everything is a process. Women, because we birth (whether it's an idea or a child), must be more aware of the process of development, the process of creation. Then we will realize that most of development, creation, and birthing is dark, behind the scenes. What we do inwardly is much more important than what we do outwardly. It's when we go inside that we really cultivate and harness our power. But where are we taught about this?

We used to have finishing schools and I think we need to have them again. Not to learn the finishing touches for our external experience, but to learn the finishing touches on the internal process of creation and birthing and development. Women have a very poor understanding of the process that enables them to claim their power. It is critically important and we are not even aware of it. For that reason, I am constantly reciting one of my favorite phrases: "trust the process." Even when you can't see it, it's happening. You just have to have faith.

Master Silence

Learn how to go within yourself, whether that's through prayer, meditation, journaling, or questioning yourself. Give yourself time to explore your internal landscape. Master silence. Shut your mouth, shut your eyes, shut your ears. Master living in silence.

Find Peace

Women have a peace within nature and with animals. It's so important for women to reconnect with the earth, each other, and animals, as well as sounds, lights, and colors. Take time for yourself. Take a bath. Spend some time alone. Listen to some music. *Yesterday I Cried* is all about me spending three days in and out of the bathtub. You can do some mighty powerful work in the bathtub.

Practical Rules

Women need to take the lessons that they learn and turn them into practical rules to be used in everyday living. Take a walk and record your thoughts. Always be present with yourself—that is the key to cultivating your personal power.

Q I think that one reason why women—especially those who work—have such a hard time letting go of the male forms of power they have been taught is that they are afraid they will not be able to succeed. They don't trust that if they are themselves and depend on their own inner strength, they won't fail.

One phrase taught me how to live in the truth of my being: God is my source and my supply. Ten years ago I put up a sign that says "I work for God, Inc." Now that has taken me into places like the legal field and publishing. But I don't work for Simon and Schuster, I work for God and I take my directions from Him. It's taken me ten years to get them to finally accept that, although they print and publish the book, I work for God.

That's a real special place to be, because what happens is our eyes cast out onto the world and we see, or our ears are attuned to the world and we hear. We start believing what we can and can't do based on what we see and hear, and these external expressions contradict one another. For example, we are taught that power is a certain type of body, that one woman is better than another based on how she looks. Women think we have to act like men but look like Barbie dolls if we're going to get ahead. Then they criticize you for being *too* Barbie. Black women don't even have anything in common with Barbie. Even the Barbies of color don't look like us. So where do we fit?

The truth is, no matter how we look on the outside, we are all capable of being expressions of feminine energy. We have a shared power and purpose: to teach, to heal, to nurture, to support, to bring beauty and love on the planet. That is the role of feminine nature. It doesn't matter if you are Jewish, Catholic, Baptist, or Episcopalian; black, white, or Native American. If you are an expression of feminine energy, you have a purpose for being here.

To me, Mother Teresa is the epitome of feminine power. Wearing a sackcloth, with no makeup or bra, she was clearly not physically attractive, but let her walk into the room and there was nothing that she could not do or have. She showed up in the fullness of her inner feminine beauty and offered who she was—true love. There was a lot of criticism of her because she was taking donations from everywhere, even the mob. And she came forth to say that, yes, she had taken money from the mob, but she didn't care. It didn't matter where it came from because she was answering to God, and not the media.

That's why you have to draw the power from the inside—because it's too contradictory on the outside. Until women get back to a really clear understanding of their purpose, the contradictions about the external world will pit woman against woman and we will continue to experience separation among ourselves. We have to learn to see the problem or the situation from a higher place in order to figure it out.

Q You often talk about listening to your heart when contemplating change. Where do we find the courage to make other choices in life?

Be true to yourself. Be true to what you hear inside. Begin within. Master the silence. Make another choice because, remember, everything we do in life is a choice. You have to accept the fact—the truth—that you are powerful. How do you do that? I don't know. You just have to accept it. It's an unfolding process, but at least say to yourself that you accept yourself. Move from that frame of mind. Move that thought into your world, into your life. From there, claim your dependence on yourself. Accept the fact that we are expressions of power, that we define power, or that we are powerful.

And observe. Be diligently aware. The power of observation for women is so critical. At all times you must observe yourself: what you are doing, feeling, thinking, saying. And once you learn how to do that, it just happens automatically. Observe yourself, and whenever you are making choices based on fear, dependence, guilt, shame, or anger, make another choice.

Take the idea of entering a meeting. Don't be driven to the meeting, be drawn to the purpose of the meeting. When you are drawn to the purpose, you go into the meeting with a vision, an internal purpose. You're not looking to give or get anything from the meeting, but you are just there, allowing it to unfold. That is a very disciplined process. When I go into a meeting, I know what I am going to do before I get there. I've already begun within. Now it may come to pass in the meeting that I have to discuss this or discuss that, but I already know where I am headed.

If someone says, "Oh, you're a difficult woman," immediately it triggers the emotional programming of: "I'm not

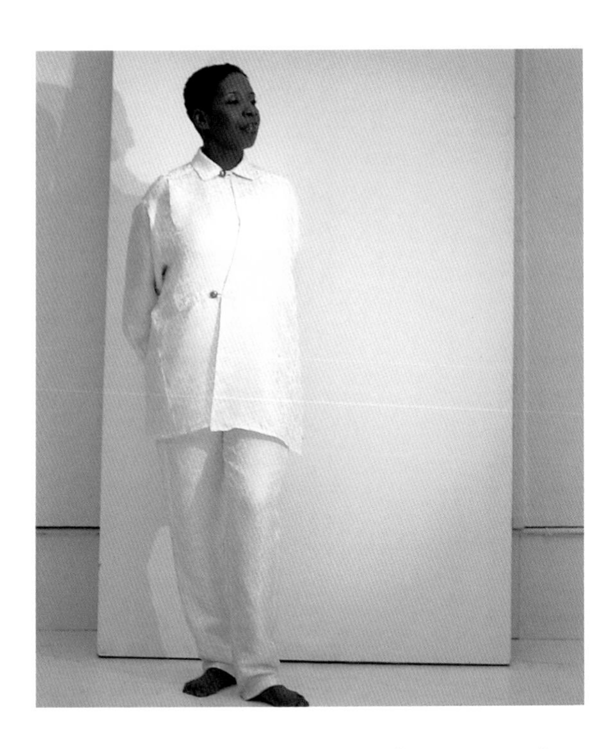

WHAT WE DO INWARDLY IS MUCH MORE IMPORTANT THAN WHAT WE DO OUTWARDLY. IT'S WHEN WE GO INSIDE THAT WE CULTIVATE AND HARNESS OUR POWER.

doing something right. There is something wrong with me. I'm not good enough." It triggers that within us. That's why I say, begin within. You've got to release the hairpin from all of those triggers so the next time that person says you're a difficult woman, you say, "You're absolutely right. You're very astute. I'm glad you noticed that." You can stand in your power and say, "Yes, I'm difficult."

Q What about our roles as mothers versus workers? The love of our children and the desire to be with them is superceded by the necessity of providing an income. This is the challenge for all working mothers.

Issues of abandonment, rejection, unimportance, valuelessness, and worthlessness all stem from parents leaving the raising of their children to others from the time that the children are very, very young. Eventually, with enough pressure from women, the powers that be will be forced to provide a workplace that is child-friendly. I believe that there's a point at which children can be lovingly separated from their mothers, usually when they're around seven years old, and moving into their second life cycle. I think it's absolutely necessary that they be given more independence at that time. They then get an opportunity to experiment with everything that their parents have already taught them. The mother's role shifts from nurturing to guidance. They can go out and when they hit somebody in the head or take someone's cookies, they get the opportunity to experience the consequences of all of the things their parents have taught them not to do at home. It's that experience that's going to help them make better choices in their lives.

When you hear women talk about how awesome motherhood is, how absolutely incredible it is, and how deep it takes them into themselves and their love, it's because they're beginning within. I want to encourage that mind-set, which is why I want to become a midwife for younger women. This movement has a lot to do with the fact that we are acknowledging that life begins early within us. With the process of in-utero teaching, a woman becomes an active mother long before the baby is born. They are conscious of what they eat and what they do and how they move. Slowly but surely women are moving away from some of the structures that men have been giving us. There are changes taking place in the hearts and minds of women that are going to rock the world. Women are changing their minds about who they are and what their role in the world order will be. They are learning to be responsible for healing their mental, physical, emotional, and spiritual selves. Women are learning to love themselves and each other. Most of all, women are evolving to the point where they are no longer willing to accept crap from themselves or anyone else. It's happening slowly, but it is happening.

IYANLA VANZANT'S SPIRITUAL POWER

Sit down, shut up, and listen. If you are busy all the time—always moving from one task to another, one experience to the next—it is quite easy to lose touch with yourself and what you need. Practicing conscious sitting will provide you with an opportunity to get a grip. Conscious sitting is like a spiritual pause: you push the pause button for a moment before you move on to the next phase of living. Sit in a quiet and comfortable place. (A bathroom stall is just fine!) Quiet the mind and body by sitting absolutely still for five minutes. Doing this several times throughout the day will allow you to experience your thoughts and feelings without having to do anything about them. Conscious sitting also enhances your powers of observation and familiarizes you with your inner voice.

Learn mindful conservation. We measure our importance in life by the number of things we are doing. We missed the lesson in conserving our resources. The greatest enemy to the principle of conservation is the fear of being lazy, stingy, and selfish. Time, money, and knowledge are all resources worthy of conserving. Spending time doing things that do not bring you or anyone else pleasure or joy is a waste of resources. Spending money in ways and on things that do not benefit you or anyone else is a waste of your resources. Trying to convince people that there is something that you know that could be beneficial to them when they are resistant to hearing you is a waste of resources. Only when we learn the value of who we are and what we are, do we become mindful of conservation. When you understand the value of your presence on the planet, you are able to give more when you do give.

Have open-heart surgery. Allow yourself to feel. Prayers open your heart to the truth of your soul. Going into your heart and allowing yourself to feel what is hidden or buried there is the most self-loving, self-affirming gift you can give yourself. When you explore, examine, and embrace your feelings, you move beyond the limitations and chatter of the mind. By sitting consciously, taking a few deep breaths, placing both hands over your heart, and allowing your mental energy to drift down to the center of your chest, you enliven the energy of your being. Gently affirm to yourself: "My heart is now open to the truth." As the feelings come up, do not question or judge them. Do not make them right or wrong, good or bad. Opening your heart daily, or at least weekly, keeps you in touch with the deepest sense of who you are.

Talk to yourself. (It's okay, people already think you're crazy.) Some of us are so out of touch with our hearts that we can no longer feel. Talk to yourself. A conscious and compassionate dialogue—the kind of dialogue that you would have with a friend or loved one who needs a shoulder to cry on. You can do this anywhere, but try finding a quiet place. Take a few deep breaths. Ask yourself simple questions such as "How are you really feeling today?" or "What do you want to do for yourself?" Once you've asked the question, respond out loud. If it shocks, surprises, or frightens you, just take a deep breath. Allow yourself to complete each sentence without thinking that it's right or wrong, and don't try to come up with answers to the problems. It may feel a little silly at first, but the more time you spend talking and listening to yourself, the more loving the relationship will become between you and you.

Play with yourself. Loosen up, girlie. Don't be so serious all the time. Remember, there is a little girl inside who needs some attention. If you don't give it to her she will act out. To keep her happy and content, you must learn to play a few hours a day for a few days a week. Have a tea party and talk to your imaginary friends. Put on a show for an imaginary audience. Get yourself a coloring book and some crayons. Give yourself a little time to do all the things you never got to do or were told not to do. If it gets really fun, invite some friends over and you can all play together. As you learn to play, you will rediscover your innocence, your sweetness, and your creative energy.

Develop compassion. Few of us have mastered what it really means to be nice. Women are natural nurturers yet we often end up resenting it. If you feel the need to jump in and save somebody for fear that if you don't they will pull you down, or if you cannot watch other people suffer because you are afraid the same thing might happen to you if you don't help, you have not reached the state of personal mastery that allows you to be compassionate. If you are acting purely from the need to be nice, you are going to end up feeling used.

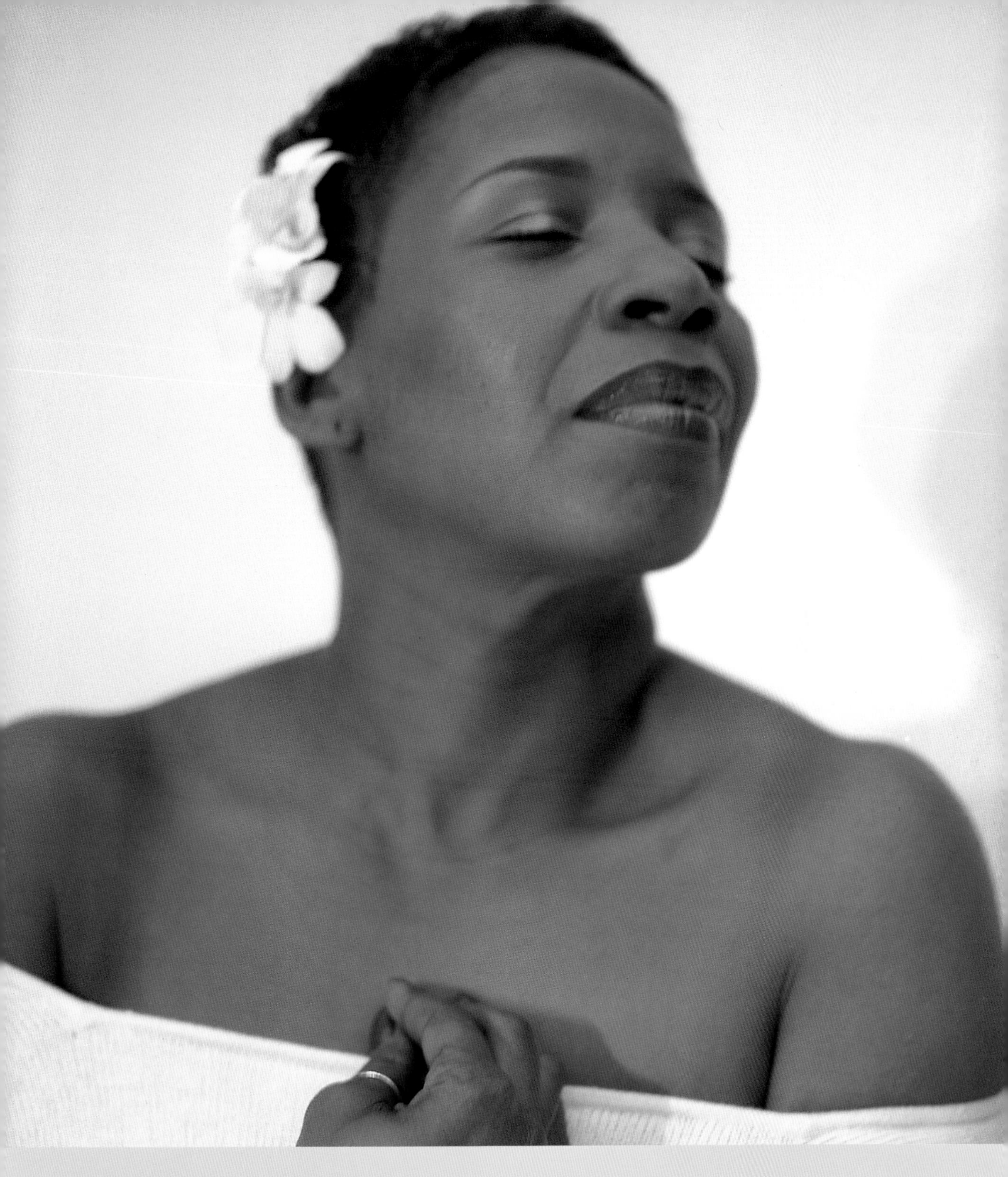

Play dead. Many of us fear death. We are afraid that we won't get to do all we want to do before we die, and then after we die, nothing will t done (even if it does, you know it won't be done right). Confront the thing you fear. Playing dead allows you to surrender yourself and your e to the divine, bringing yourself face to face with the reality that life moves through you no matter what you tell yourself. On a hard surface ke the floor), lie still with your eyes closed. Become aware of your breath. Listen to yourself inhale and exhale. Feel your heart beating. Allow e to pass through you and around you without moving or responding to any thoughts, feelings, or interruptions. Playing dead at least once nonth will help you get a clearer idea of how you choose to live.

DREW BARRYMORE

Actress Drew Barrymore is living proof that someone can survive "too much too soon." She landed her first acting role at eleven months and at age six she became famous for her role in *E.T.*, one of the most popular films in movie history. But by age nine Drew was an alcoholic. She recounted her experience of sadness, pain, and a bad family history in *Little Girl Lost* after a successful rehab stay at age fourteen. Today, at the age of twenty-four, Drew is one of the most sought-after actors in Hollywood and a role model for young girls. She has her own successful production company, Flower Films, with partner and old friend Nancy Juvonen. A dedicated philanthropist, Drew donates her time and resources to a number of charities, including the Female Health Foundation and the Wildlife Waystation.

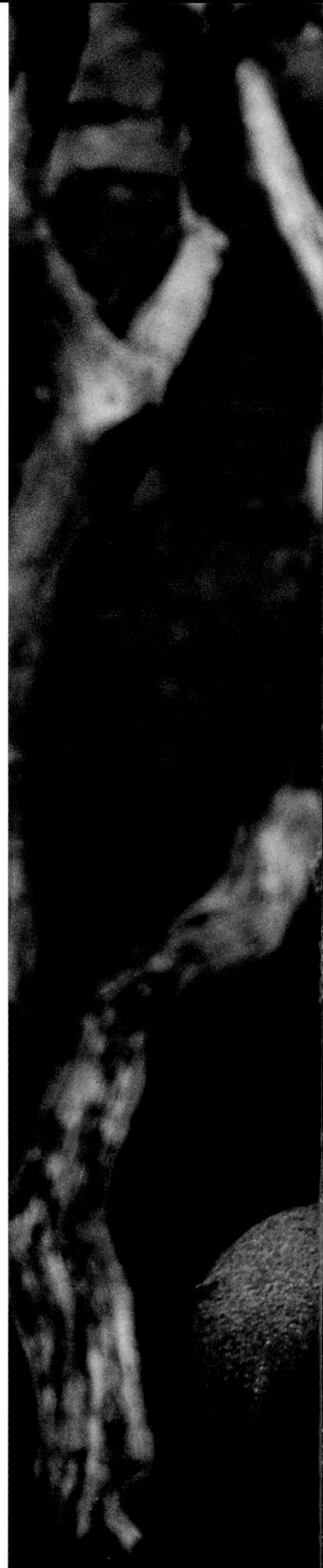

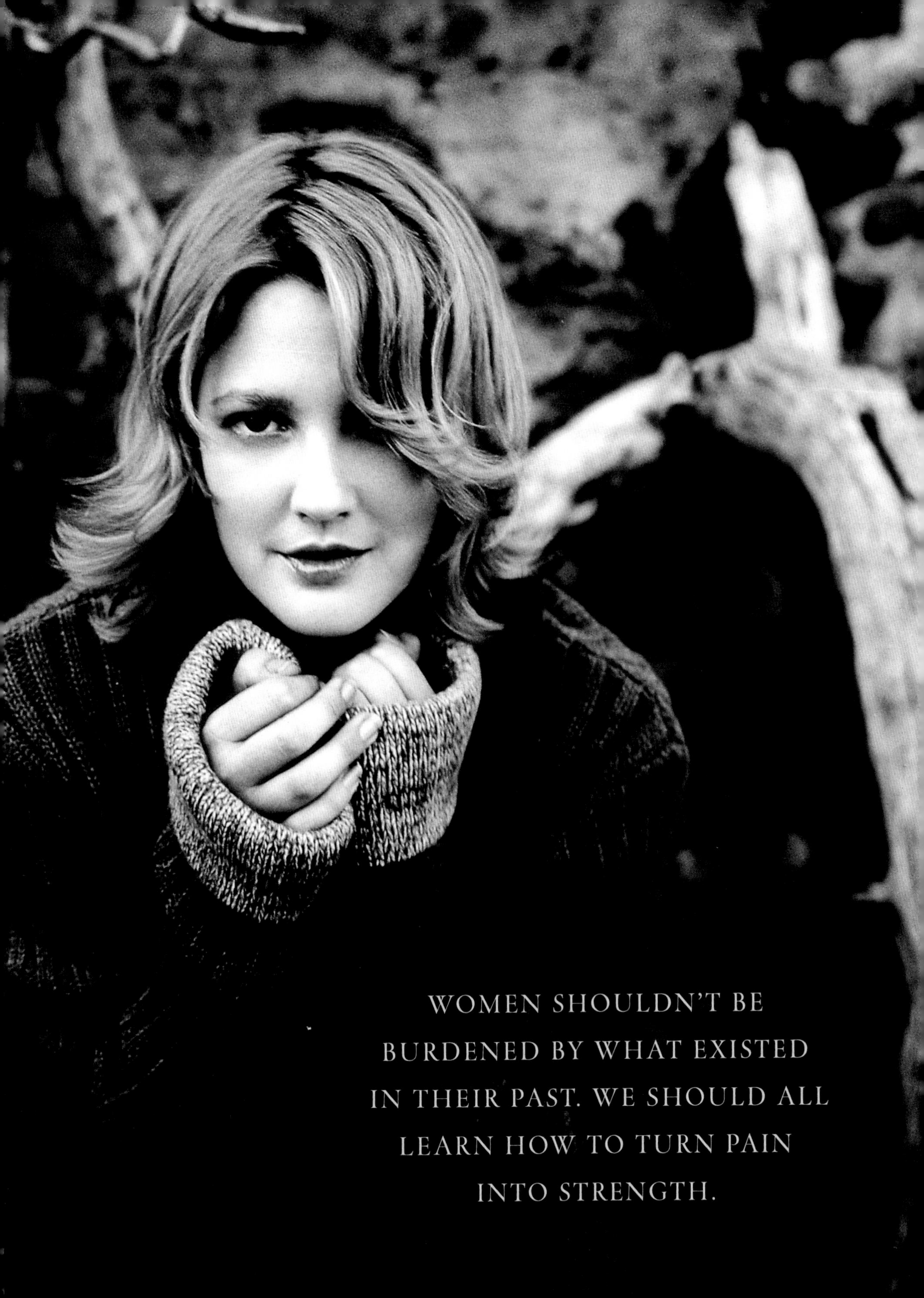
WOMEN SHOULDN'T BE
BURDENED BY WHAT EXISTED
IN THEIR PAST. WE SHOULD ALL
LEARN HOW TO TURN PAIN
INTO STRENGTH.

Q You have really reinvented your image since you overcame your addiction. What motivates you to stay on track?

It feels great to be given a second chance and I never take it for granted. I am motivated by the idea of being an inspiration to others. I certainly try to step up to bat now. I always want to be there when my friends need me. I always want to be reliable.

If you are going to go through hell, I suggest that you come back learning something. I have learned that hardships can be beneficial. Life doesn't ever give you what you can't handle. The pain I have felt in life has made me more empathetic. It has made me want to help other women heal.

I also think that the idea of reincarnation or an afterlife is a good motivator. There's a quote that says, "My bags are waiting in the next life, and I want to pack good things in those bags."

Q Could you offer any insight into self-discovery? What rules do you live by that have helped you to develop such grace and dignity?

If you are passionate about something in life, be nice about it. Because if you yell, you're only going to make someone feel bad and you're going to hate yourself later. I have a great deal of hunger and fervor, but I won't push anyone to the side to get where I'm going. I want to create my own road. I never want to get to the point where it's all about my needs and to hell with everybody. When I'm on the set I treat everyone with the same respect.

I've also learned that you don't have to stress to do a good job. Women tend to be hypercritical of themselves because of the double standards surrounding us. In all of the work that we do in life—whether it's being a full-time mom or CEO—there is a certain amount of passion and enthusiasm required to do a good job. I realized after the filming of *Ever After* that if I had the same level of enthusiasm without the stress, self-deprecation, and constant self-criticism, I still would have been successful. I battle with myself in my head all the time, but each year I get better. I used to look in the mirror and feel shame; now I feel pride.

There are so many pressures that are put upon young women today. I want to do whatever I can to help alleviate that and help them feel beautiful inside, which is the only beauty there truly is. I want them to look upon the movies that I make as medicine. As an actor I'll continue to do darker characters, but I always want to have the opportunity to make movies that have terrific positivity.

Ego Mania

When ego rules your soul, you are cut off from the possibilities of a fabulous life. Beware of the need to be right and know when NOT to have the last word.

To Err Is Human

Even if you fall on your face, you can pull yourself back together. Disregard the shame and embarrassment and remember that what looks like a mistake on the outside is often a deliberate signal of a much-needed change.

Courage

Allow yourself to recognize your own tendencies of anger, greed, fear, jealousy, and selfishness. When you become aware of these habits, you can then begin to change them. This takes courage because it begins with looking at yourself as you are.

Q You really are self-made. You have come so far with your positive attitude and smart business sense.

That's true, but ironically it wasn't until recently that I realized how important my relationship with myself is. At times in my life I felt abandoned not only by my family and friends, but also by myself. I always hoped that I would find someone who would make me feel like they weren't going to leave me. I pictured that person to be a silhouette of someone larger—I never thought that it could be me. This has been an amazing revelation that I never thought could be true. It's changed my life. It makes me wake up differently. For the first time in my life, I realize that great happiness doesn't only have to come from being involved with someone.

Before, I think I lacked independence. I really liked doing things with people, but I think that there was also a real safety in that for me. Now I think of the time that I spend with others as a gift rather than a need. We all need people but I never realized what a decent companion I am to myself. I've never done so much alone before. A while ago I went to Hawaii by myself, and I go on solo excursions all the time, even if it's just a walk around the block. When you've looked to others for happiness for years and years, it's great to realize that you can give yourself that feeling. It's all about living life one day at a time and appreciating all of the experiences that come along with it, good or bad. If you're going to be alive on this planet, you have to suck the marrow out of every day and get the most out of it. I think that life is a series of learning experiences. It's full of questions. And when you find the answers to some of them it's so fulfilling.

Q **What has it been like, as a woman at the age of twenty-four, to start your own production company and compete with Hollywood?**

People ask me what kind of difficulties I have had as a woman in my industry. The truth is that I don't believe other people are responsible for what happens to us; only we can determine the outcome of our experiences. I think I have put bigger barriers in my way than anyone in the business has. I have had tremendous opportunities. People give me a lot of time and respect. They trust me with their money, and I feel heard. I don't have any complaints. Not one.

I'M ALWAYS TRYING NOT TO BE SO HARD ON MYSELF. I DON'T FEEL ANY AWKWARDNESS OR BITTERNESS TOWARD MY LIFE.

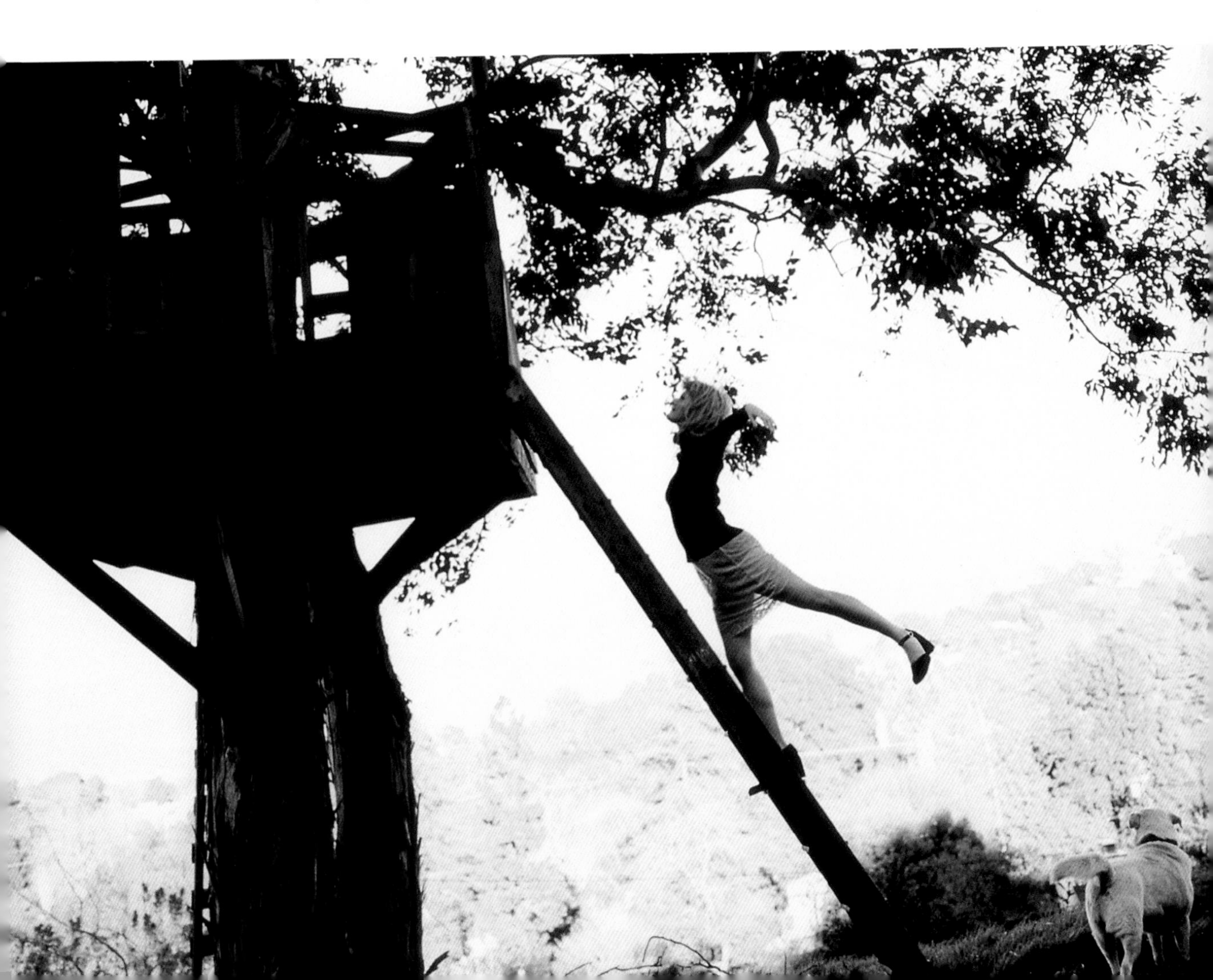

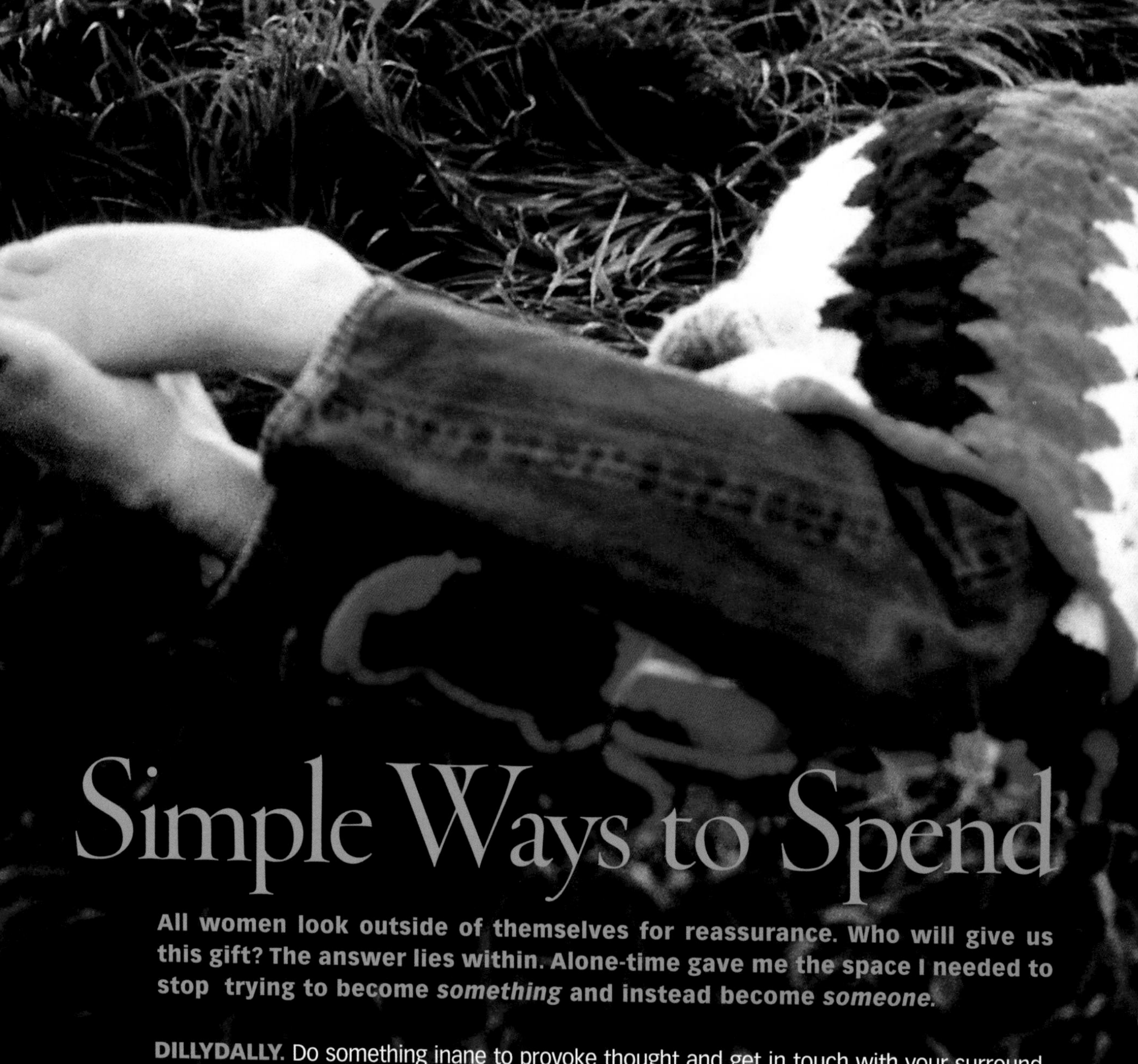

Simple Ways to Spend

All women look outside of themselves for reassurance. Who will give us this gift? The answer lies within. Alone-time gave me the space I needed to stop trying to become *something* and instead become *someone*.

DILLYDALLY. Do something inane to provoke thought and get in touch with your surroundings. To feel alive is to be able to see and hear and look. Try to stay in the present with your thoughts. I really believe that life happens in moments—each one to be valued in its own way. A slow walk can help you discover places or thoughts you might otherwise have missed.

ESCAPE. Always waiting for a travel partner? Forget it. Search a travel guide for the destination of your choice and hit the road. Bask in the glory of your unaccountability and relax. Reflective qualities of a getaway for one can be life-altering.

TAKE A NAP. A lot of my best ideas and revelations come to me in my dreams. This is true for all of us, but we need to unclutter our minds in order for them to create.

DINNER FOR ONE. Some people think that there is nothing sadder than a solitary dinner. On the contrary, dinner and a movie (of your choice!) for one can be just the ticket. Whether you're having macaroni and cheese (my favorite) or truffle fois gras, enjoy the fact that you can savor the meal without the risk of talking with your mouth full.

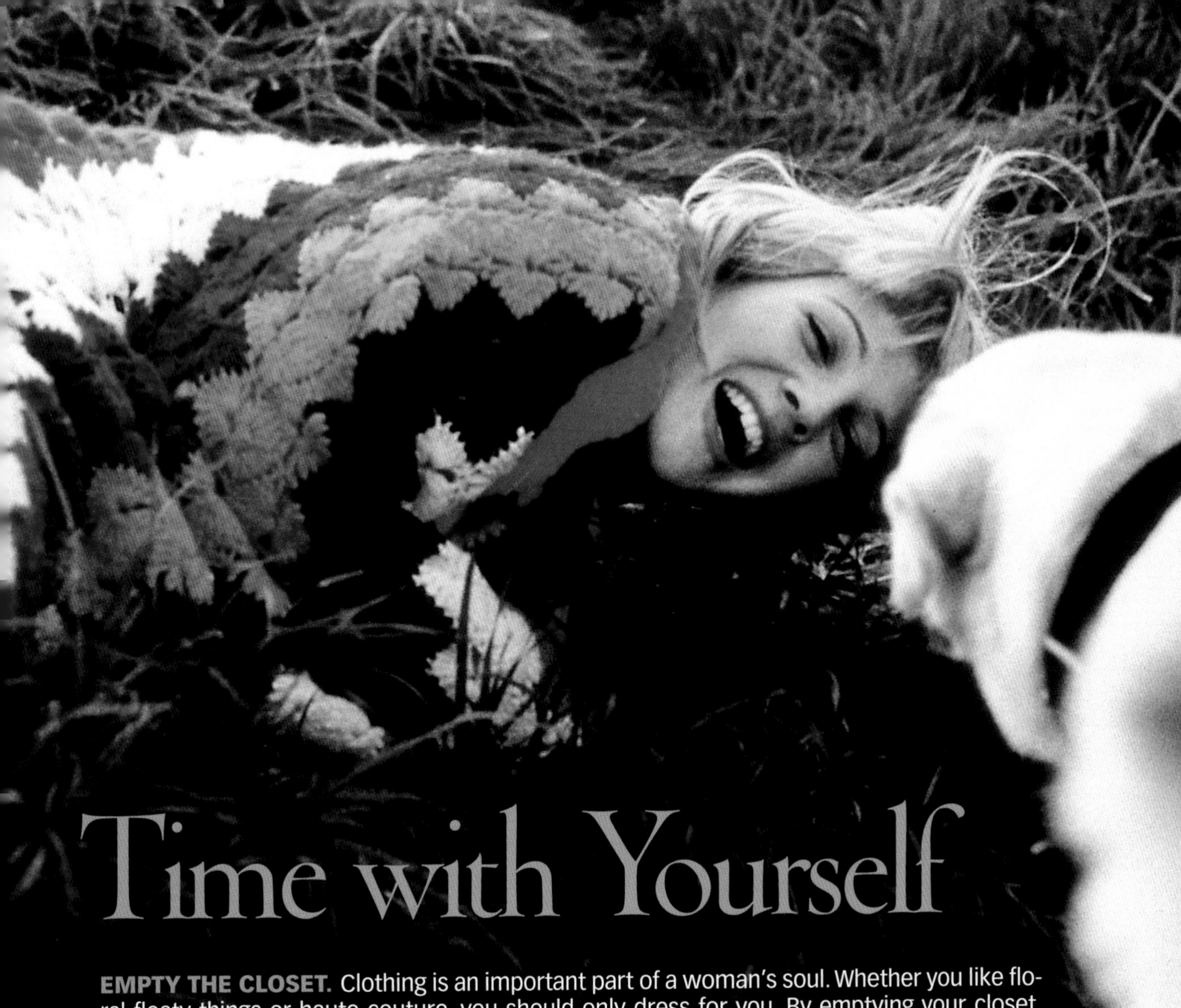

Time with Yourself

EMPTY THE CLOSET. Clothing is an important part of a woman's soul. Whether you like floral floaty things or haute couture, you should only dress for you. By emptying your closet, literally, you can begin to investigate the connection between your personal style and your sense of self. Every article of clothing that we own has its own story. Do your clothes really reflect who you are? Maybe it's time to release some old baggage and make a few purchases that make you feel beautiful inside and out.

INDULGE IN NATURE. Lie in a field, adopt a tree, start a garden, or plant a few seeds in a pot on your windowsill. There is nothing as peaceful as enjoying nature or nurturing it and watching it grow. When I was a little girl my home life was less than perfect. When things got rough I would head out to our avocado tree with the salt shaker and a spoon, sit on my swing, and eat one avocado after another. I think that's why I was such a chubby child, but I loved that tree. I hugged it every day. Today, my fruit trees are the things that make me the happiest at my new home.

TAKE LONG DRIVES. I love to take long drives and stick my head out the window like a dog. Pack up your favorite music and some snacks and let the spirit move you wherever that may be. Bring along a map and you might make a few discoveries.

FEELING FRAZZLED? TAKE A BATH. Let the water run while you soak. After twenty

SHARON GANNON

Sharon Gannon is the cofounder of New York's Jivamukti Yoga Center, **which is renowned for its vigorous physical workouts and strong foundation in the ancient yogic texts, as well** as for its celebrity clientele. To her yoga students, Sharon brings a rare blend of scholarly knowledge, artistry, and a highly disciplined asana and meditation practice. She is also an animal-rights activist and the author of *Cats and Dogs Are People Too!*, which looks at the insensitive attitudes that result in cruelty to animals and offers optimistic measures to improve our relationships with other species. Sharon acknowledges the great gift she has received from her gurus Pattabhi Jois, Brahmananda Sarasvati, and Swami Nirmalananda.

Q In everyone's life there is a pivotal moment of truth, a loss of innocence. This moment is instrumental in shaping our future. For me it was the realization that nothing lasts forever. I wanted to save time in a bottle, document history. What life moment made you decide to become involved in spiritual leadership?

That question brings back a memory that I haven't thought of for years. I can already feel myself starting to cry. When I was a little girl my parents lived a fly-by-night lifestyle. My stepfather drank a lot and they weren't very centered. One day, I was in the backyard with him. He was drunk and decided to shoot squirrels for fun. He laid their dead bodies out on the picnic table. I had no idea they were dead so I picked them up and cuddled them. My mother came out, pointed at me, and started to laugh. They were both laughing at me and I didn't know why. I looked down and realized that my dress was covered in blood. In that moment I realized something was wrong with them. I am still astonished that they would ridicule their own daughter's naivete.

That experience destroyed all the trust I had in my stepfather. I wasn't angry with him, but I made an about-face and began to look elsewhere for guidance. I began to realize that a person's lack of self-esteem leads to cruelty and violence. My father was a violent man. There were times when I just felt sorry for him. I realized he was uncomfortable with himself, which led to his need make other people feel uncomfortable. This lack of self-

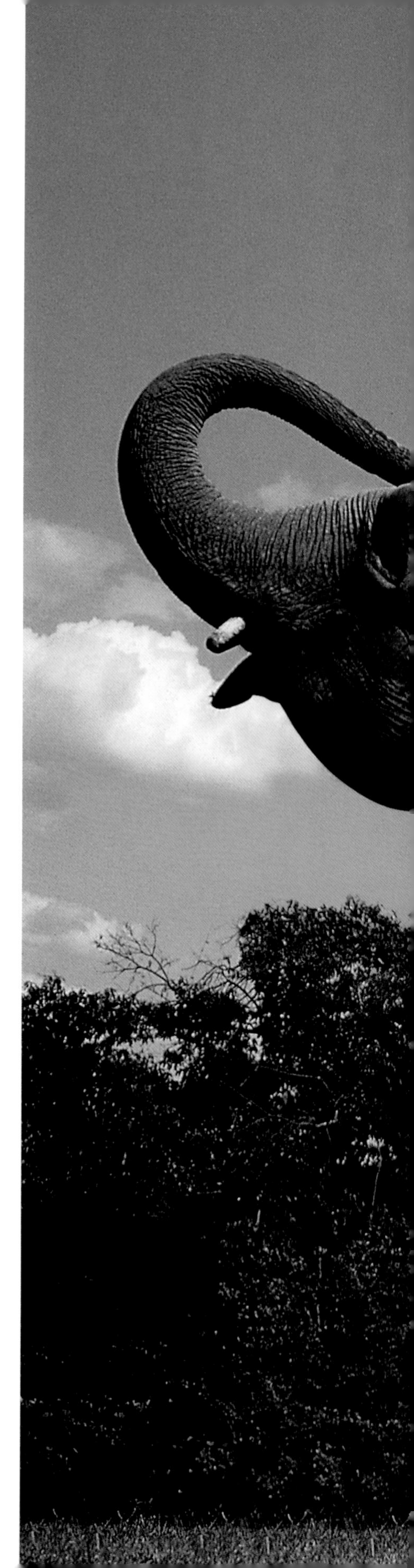

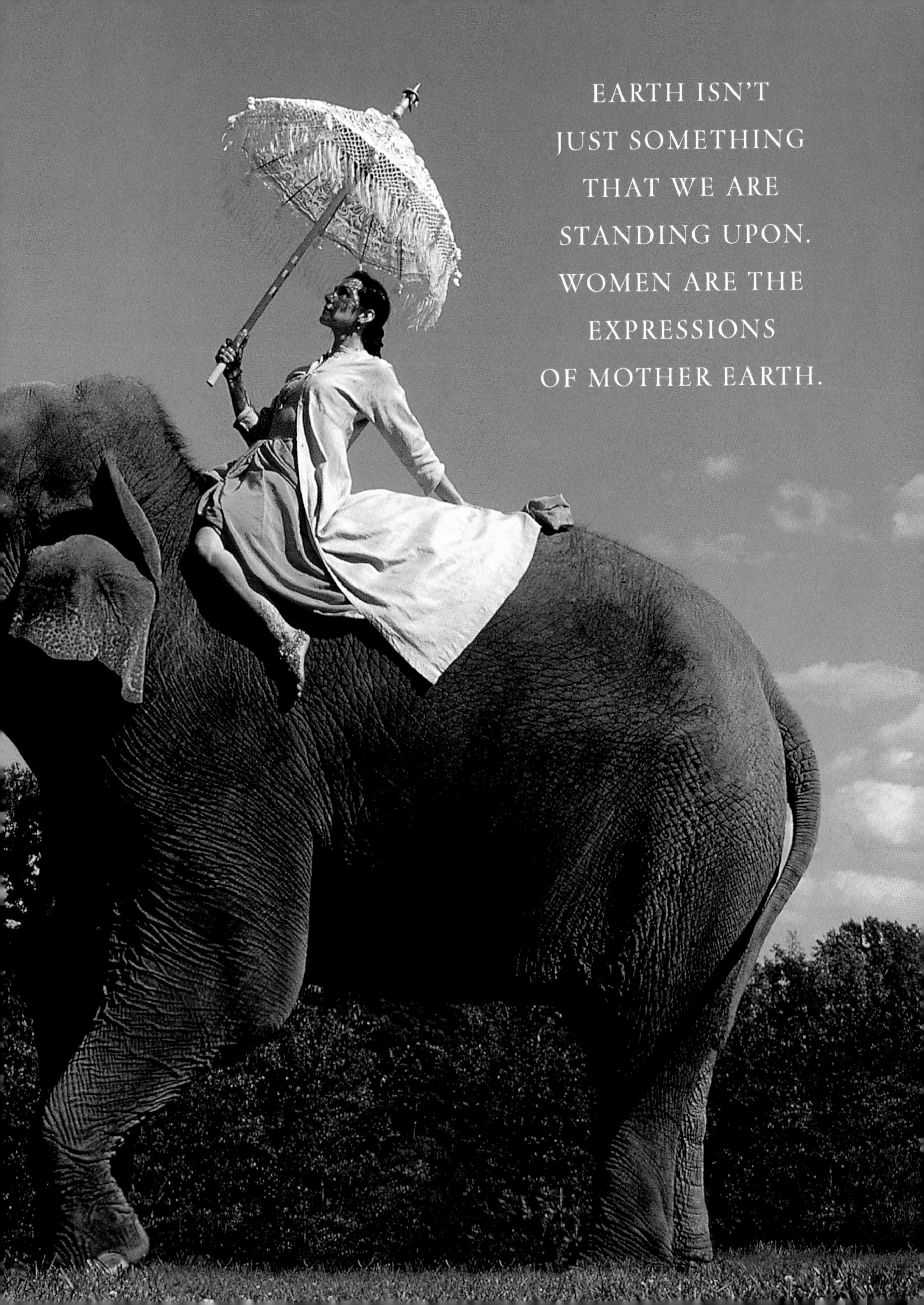

EARTH ISN'T
JUST SOMETHING
THAT WE ARE
STANDING UPON.
WOMEN ARE THE
EXPRESSIONS
OF MOTHER EARTH.

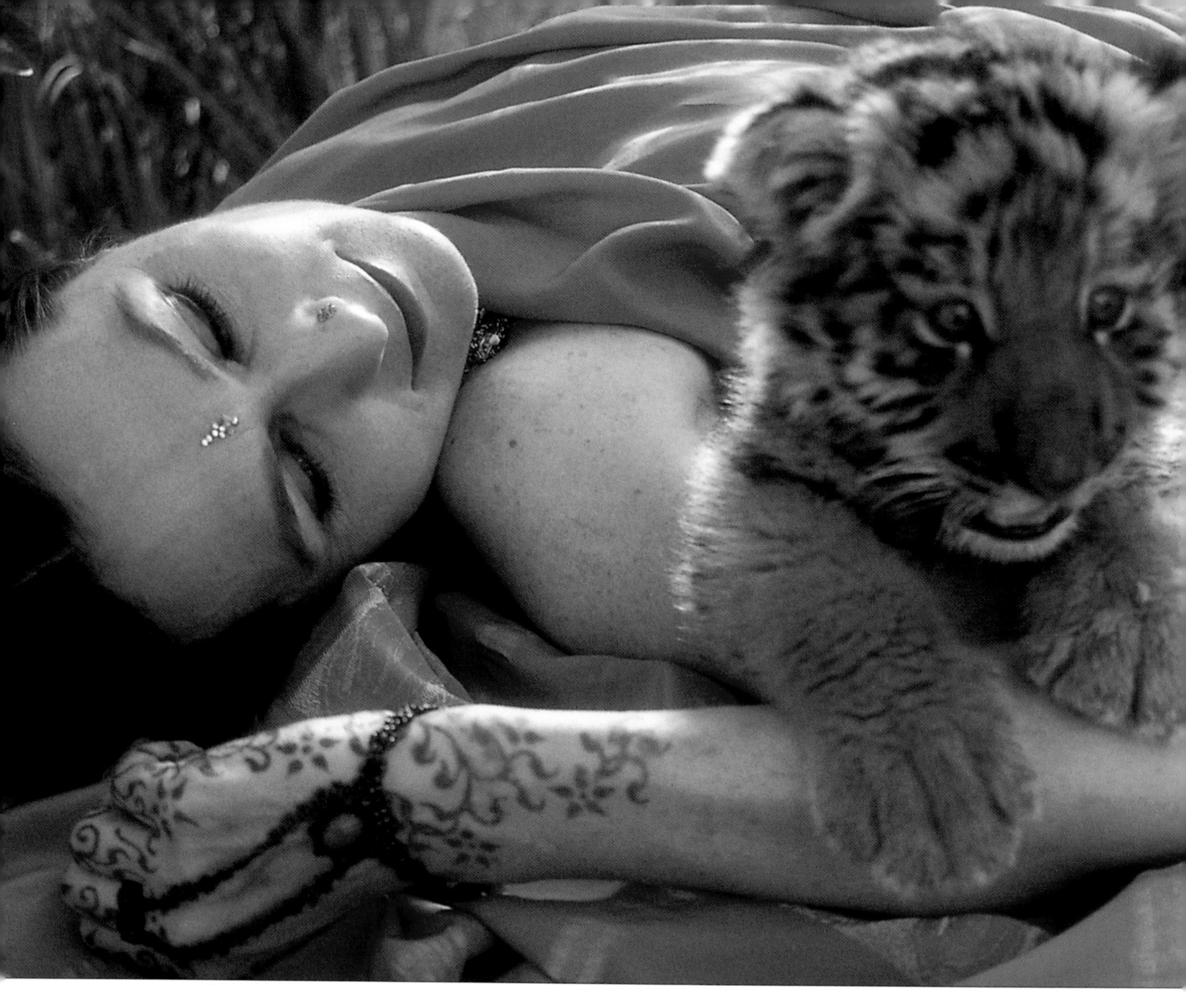

confidence is at the base of our human condition. Here in America it is manifested in the need for power and suppressing others: we treat animals and other people unkindly. This makes us feel good about ourselves. But that confidence is fleeting. We need to repeat the behavior again and again to maintain that confidence. It leaves us without any peace.

Q Westerners are readily embracing Eastern concepts, searching for a new spirituality. Why do you think this is happening?

We're well aware of the temporary value of material things that so much of Western success is based on, and we want to experience something deeper. Yoga does not dictate, "you must do asanas or suffer," because it has to be done with desire to connect to the eternal. If you have that, you're already 90 percent there. And it's a personal journey. We're not going to manipulate you into a saint.

Q We often hear the advice that we should love ourselves as we are and love others for who they are: see the best in everyone. What does yoga philosophy say about self-judgment and the judgment of others? Should we never be critical of ourselves or anyone else?

It's not so black and white. It is important to develop a discriminating eye. Meditation and yoga allow you to experience a deeper level of identity–identifying others based not on an intellectual concept of looks, wealth, or racial background, but on actual experience that can't even be defined in words. Yoga philosophy discriminates based on the question, "How is this association or situation going to get me closer to God or connect me to my source and get

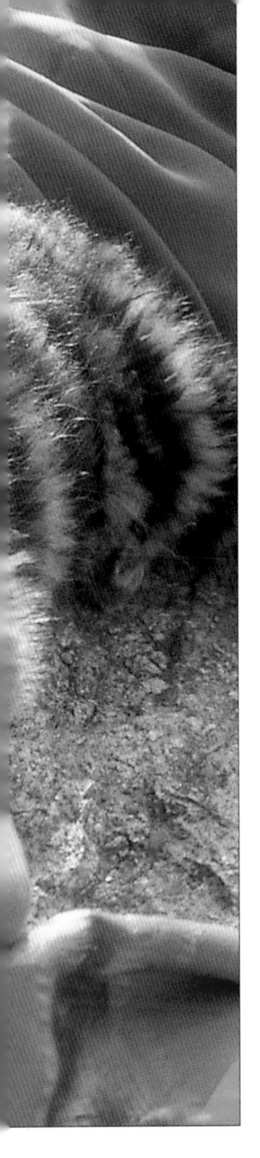

me closer to my divine potential?" Yoga leads you to see your own true, eternal self and that in others because of a deeper, divine knowledge no longer defined by other peoples' perceptions but rather by whether or not you or others are living the true, eternal self: living in bliss.

Q Visionaries like the great Dalai Lama say that the very purpose of our lives is to seek happiness. But many women who appear successful are actually very depressed. They don't know what makes them truly happy. So what is happiness?

Women tend to look to material goods to make themselves happy. Is happiness buying a new car? Affording the latest style? Getting a new haircut? If we look at the way women were regarded historically, defining happiness like this makes sense. Women were property. We had nothing of our own. Laws and rights didn't even apply to us, only to men. Today we feel successful because we are able to have things of our own. But tendencies toward materialism left by these historical scars do not lead us to true happiness. They are empty and temporary. Happiness is based on kindness and compassion. It is a state of mind. Whenever you encounter another, don't cause them harm. This is the way to real happiness. It comes from within.

Q Could you elaborate on why the ancient spiritual practice of yoga is so pertinent today?

Yoga is about connecting to the eternal source, which is the same for humans today as it was thousands of years ago. We women are suffering from the same things we have always suffered from: feeling isolated, suppressed, and disrespected. Yoga is not about being told what to do and think or being convinced that it is the teaching you should follow. It is about having the experience. We are too often watching life through TV or movies; yoga is a participation in life. By sitting quietly and attending to your breath, the source of life, you free the consciousness and become connected to God, our source of unconditional love. If practiced consistently, you can learn how to direct the flow of energy all the way down to a cellular level, so the body and mind become less susceptible to being manipulated by destructive external stimulants like stress. Think of when you are in traffic, overworked, angry, or depressed. You are affected physically and emotionally. Muscles are tight, cells are restricted, and your mind is focused on negative thoughts. Yoga and meditation release stress by allowing energy to flow again. When you attempt yoga postures, you become aware of holding stress, emotion, depression, and negativity. By moving through the positions, breathing full breaths, you release this holding, this stress. And this actually helps slow the aging process because stress is a primary factor in aging.

Q So many people live for the day when they will have enough money to do what they want. Others believe you should do what you love and the money will follow. How can the practices of yoga help us to gain perspective on our financial situation?

Yoga philosophy envisions money as a form of energy. We go shopping or out to dinner and enjoy the flow of the energy, of money. Through enjoying this exchange we become free and independent, unattached to holding. Life becomes more fun, more playful. As people become older they lose the ability to play. They are bogged down, so heavy with seriousness. At thirty years old they're already so tired they don't look forward to the next day.

Money is also about eligibility. In yoga philosophy, reality has many different levels. The first level is survival: food, shelter, and clothing. In order to learn the teachings of yoga, you must have attained this first level. You have to be eligible on the material level before you can evolve further spiritually. Put another way, you have to have a roof over your head and food to eat and then you can meditate. This was a lesson taught by the great teacher Gersha. If he knew someone was poor, he would charge $50 to teach them. If he knew someone was well off, he would charge $5. Why? The person who was poor had to do their groundwork, figure out ways to make the money, to generate energy. That in itself is spiritual evolution. Those people who thought $50 was for rich people perceived themselves as impoverished, as victims. And how can self-perceived victims perceive themselves as the Divine? Those people are not ready to receive the teachings.

Q Women today work tirelessly to have it all: motherhood, demanding careers, and an identity separate from traditional mother and wife. But most of us still feel empty and inadequate. Why, at a time when we can finally have it all, are women in such a state of dissatisfaction?

Greed. Success is based on power, wealth, and manipulation, which are attained by being greedy and selfish. Men tend toward this naturally. It begins with their physical state. A man's reproductive organs are outside of his body, making him vulnerable. This vulnerability breeds insecurity, which manifests itself in the quest for dominance and suppression. Acts of generosity and selflessness are thought of as weaknesses. Conversely, women's reproductive organs are inside the body and naturally protected. Our strengths are selflessness, generosity, and creation. But women have been drawn into the male way of perceiving success and accomplishment. We have learned to hate and disrespect our female strengths. This hateful mentality reaches deep into our lives. We learn disrespect for our own creators—our parents—with whom so many women have problems. This manifests itself in the myriad problems women have with their bodies. We physically hold shame just because we've been born women. And we focus these negative feelings primarily on our mother because we were born through her. Yoga is physiotherapy. Yoga postures—asanas—transform our hatred toward the earth, which is defined as every living being, every organic manifestation, to respect. They ground us. The word *asana* means "seat,"—the seat or position taken to strengthen our relationship to the earth and rejoice in its creation. In order to hold a pose, you must let go of the competitive, selfish mentality and instead embrace an attitude of openness, selflessness, and generosity. When attempting to stand on one leg, lift the other, and maintain your balance, you cannot think, "I will overcome my body, I will manipulate and force it." You must liberate yourself. You must rely on feminine attributes like passivity, patience, generosity, and endurance to accomplish and experience the power of asana. Through these experiences, you find power where before you saw weakness. You learn the deep satisfaction of embodying these feminine strengths, of being woman.

WHEN YOU FIND SPIRITUAL CONFIDENCE WITHIN YOURSELF, YOU ARE THEN ABLE TO BECOME AN INSTRUMENT FOR PEACE AND COMPASSION.

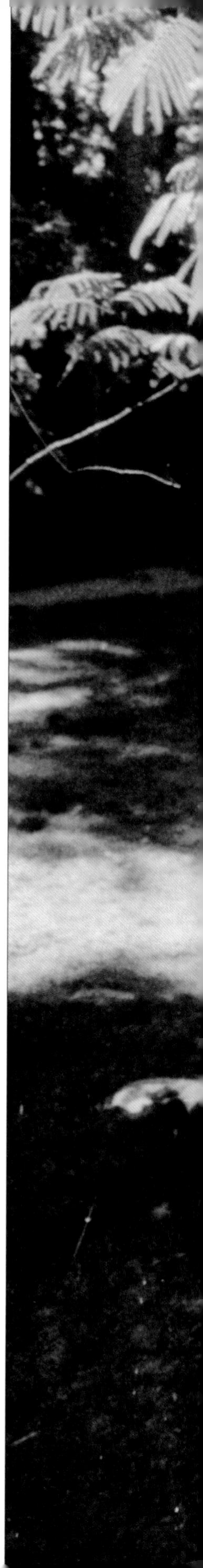

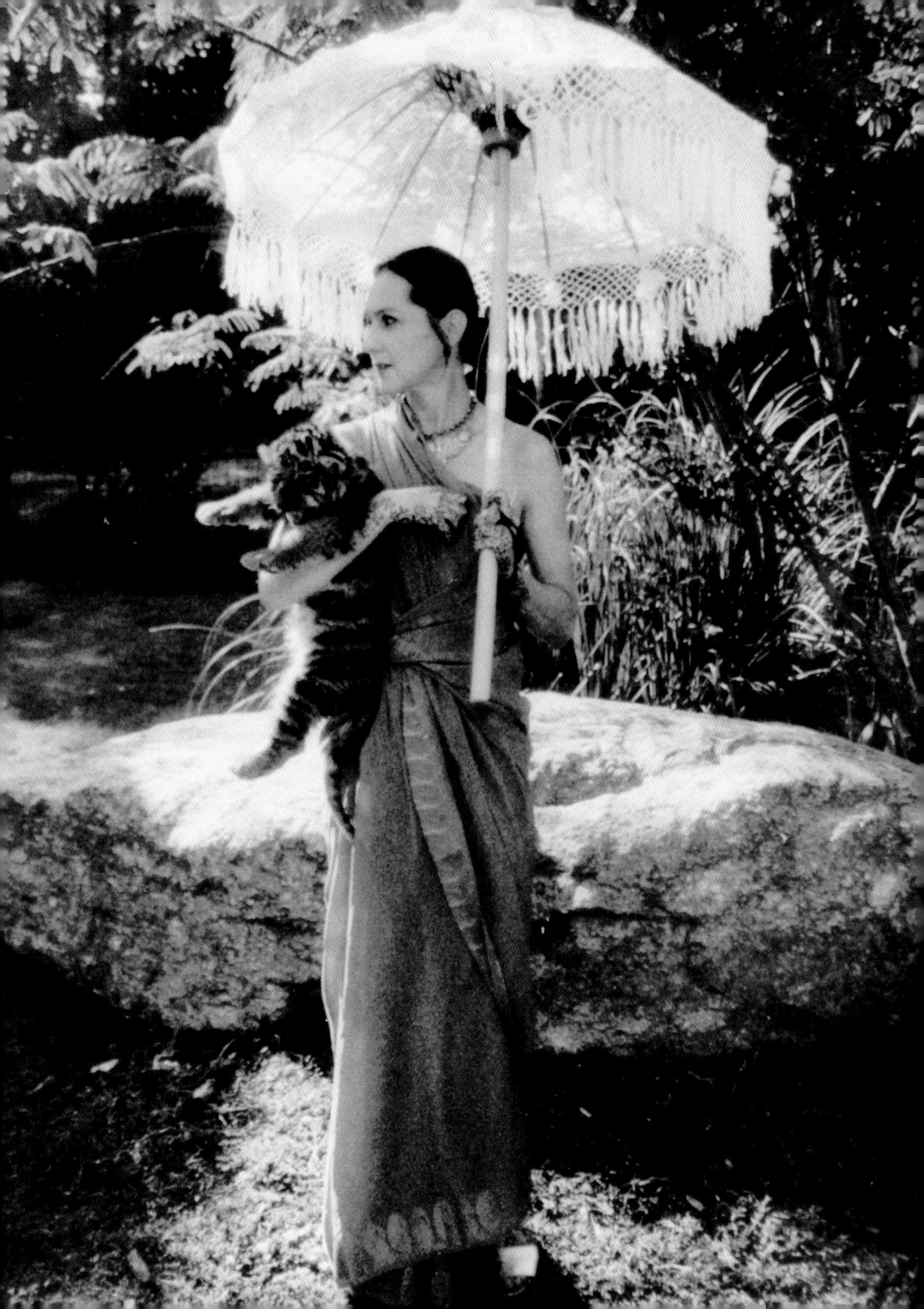

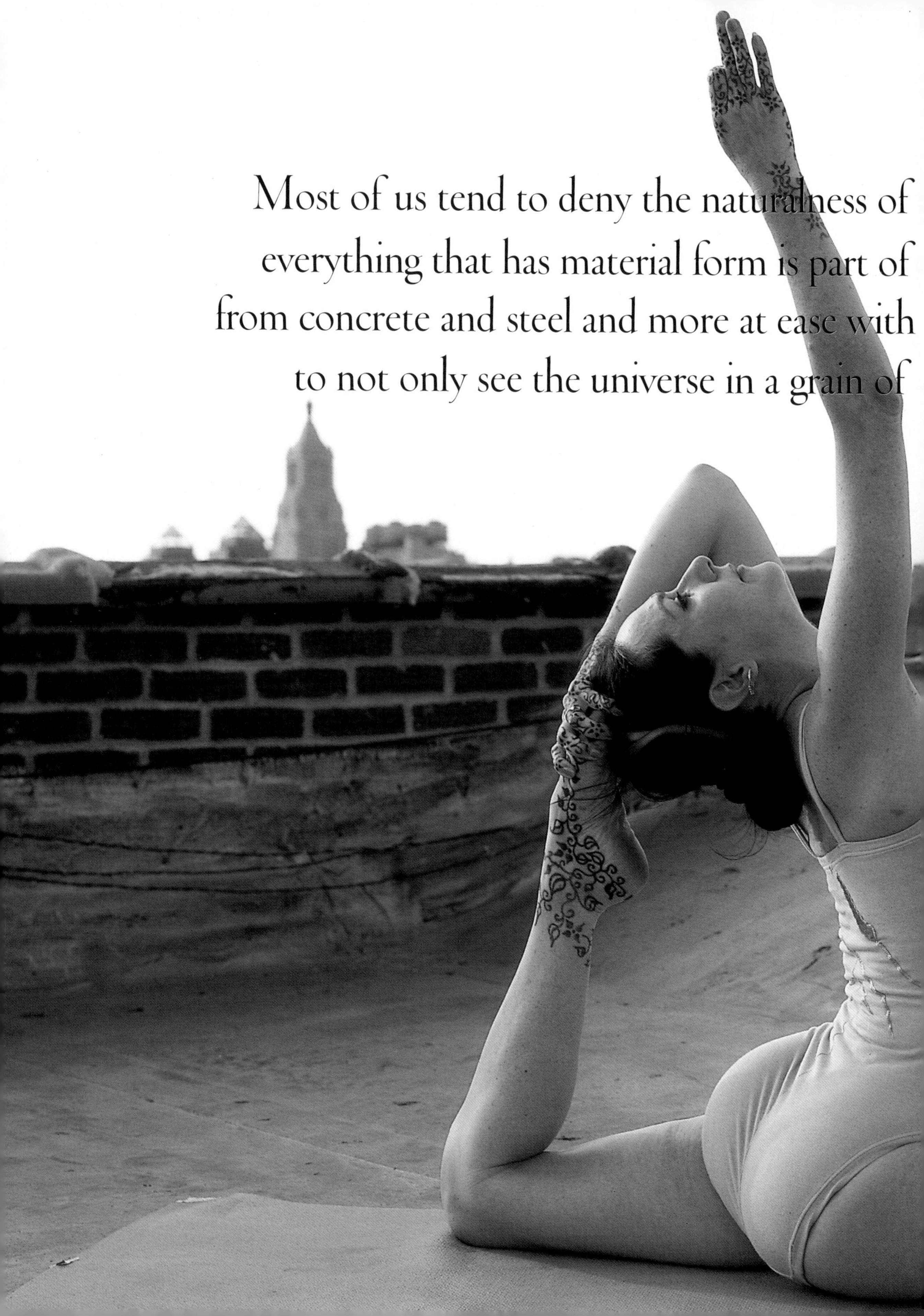

Most of us tend to deny the naturalness of
everything that has material form is part of
from concrete and steel and more at ease with
to not only see the universe in a grain of

he city, especially a city like New York, but
he divine creation. It is easy to feel separate
grass and trees. The yogi takes the challenge
sand but God in the face of the garbage man.

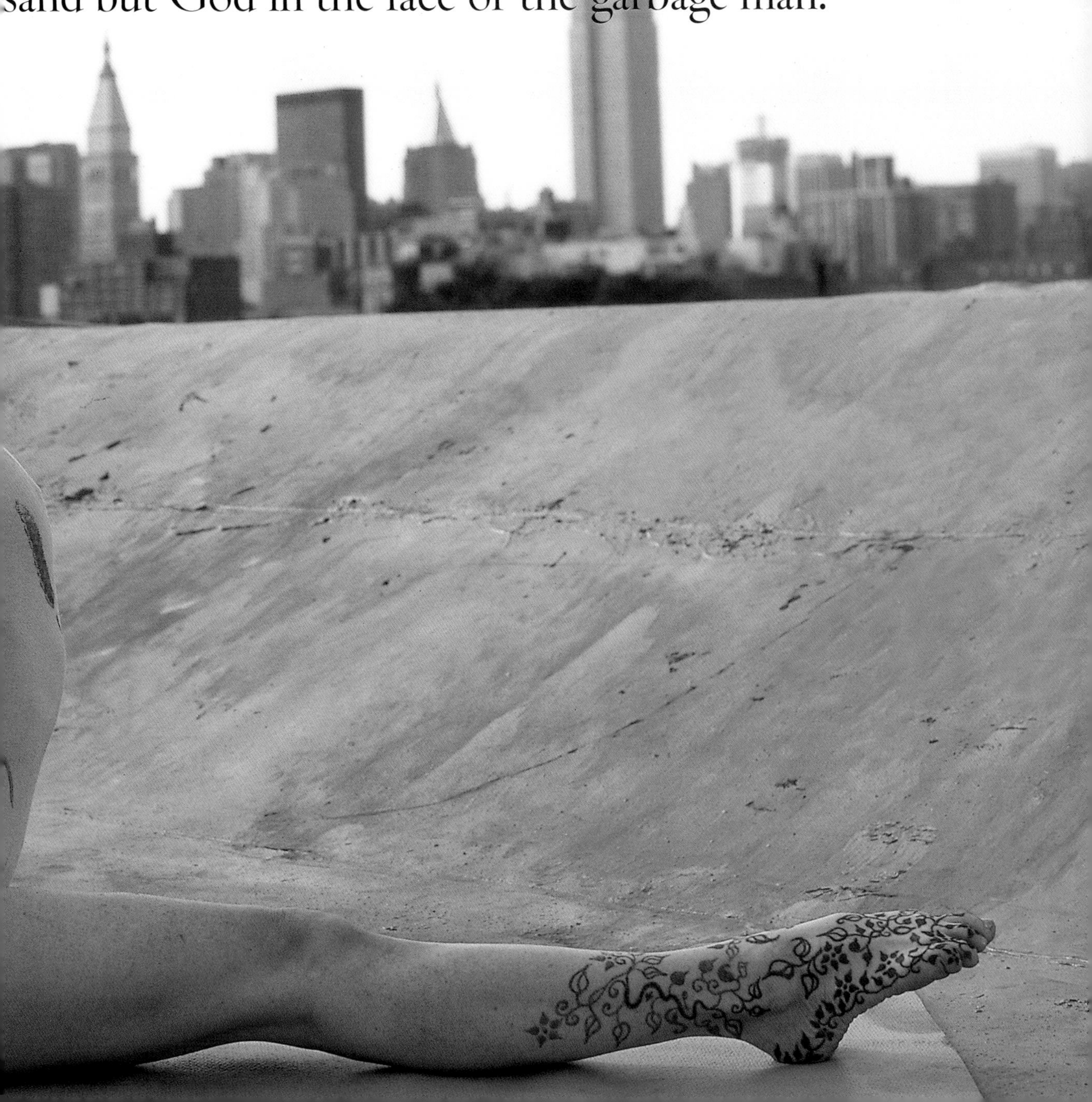

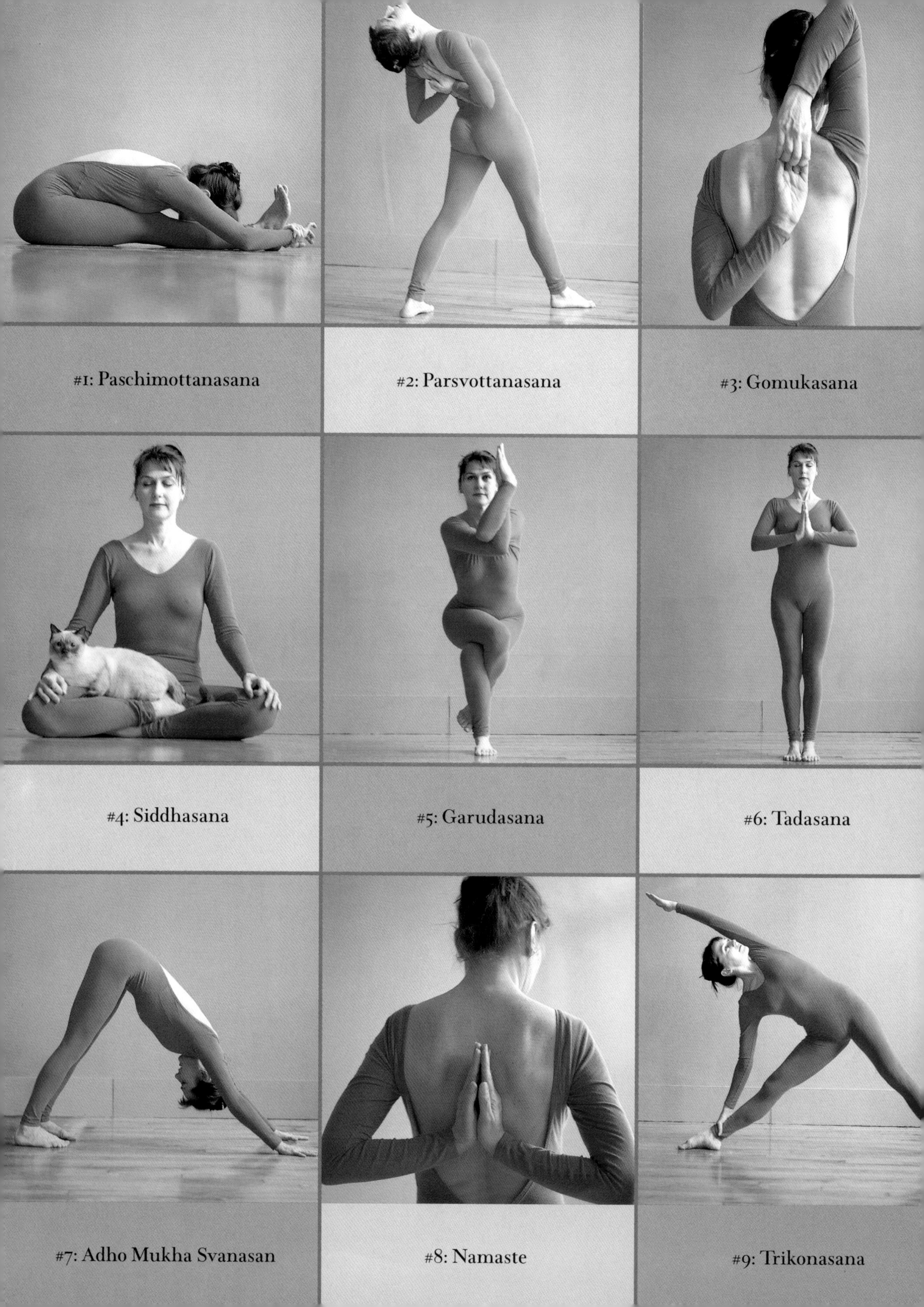

#1: Paschimottanasana

#2: Parsvottanasana

#3: Gomukasana

#4: Siddhasana

#5: Garudasana

#6: Tadasana

#7: Adho Mukha Svanasan

#8: Namaste

#9: Trikonasana

YOGA BASICS

Most people in our time, when they think of yoga, think of the various hatha yoga postures. *Asana* is the word in Sanskrit for these postures. The practice of asana really means the practice of refining one's connection to the earth and all of her beings and things. Through the practice of yoga asanas, you become strong–physically, psychologically, and spiritually. What that means is that you develop yourself to become an instrument for peace and compassion, a being who gives back instead of only taking from the earth. The practice of yoga asanas makes the yogi strong and self-confident–a confidence that comes from connecting to the innermost part of being, the heart that beats eternally in all.

#1 Paschimottanasana: The common name for this pose is seated forward bend. By actively stretching the upper body over the lower body, you will elongate the back of the spine as well as extend the front of the spine. Pull the front thighs up toward the pelvis and extend the backs of the legs actively into the floor. Do not allow the legs to relax. Feet should be flexed and parallel to each other. Breathe for five to twenty slow, steady breaths. Move deeper into this pose on exhalation. This pose stimulates digestion and helps to reduce fat in the abdominal region.

#2 Parsvottanasana: Separate the legs about three feet and turn the back foot in slightly. Grounding the feet firmly into the floor, extend both legs upward. Lift the upper chest and arch the upper spine backward. Be careful not to crunch the neck by dropping the head back; instead, lift the chest and lengthen the neck like a swan. Hold for five slow, deep breaths. This pose charges the legs with energy and brings flexibility to the hips. The backward bend stretches and oxygenates the abdominal organs.

#3 Gomukasana: *Gomuk* means "cow-face." This pose is great for practicing deep breathing. Many of us have sunken chests, a result of shallow breathing that may have a psychological origin in low self-esteem. This pose allows for full expansion of the chest. As breathing capacity increases, so does vitality and self-confidence. Stiff shoulder joints are lubricated and made more mobile. Hold for five to ten slow, full, steady breaths and then change sides.

#4 Siddhasana: (the adept's pose—variation with cat sitting on lap): This is one of the best poses for the practice of meditation. Draw your left foot in to your pelvis. Place your right leg on top of your left and tuck the right toes in between the thigh and calf of the left leg. Sit on a firm pillow if it helps to keep the back straight. Rest your hands on the knees or thighs, joining the thumb and tip of the forefinger together lightly. Cats have a strong ability to ground emotional energy, allowing you to move quite easily into deep states of meditative calm.

#5 Garudasana: This is the eagle pose (*garuda* means "eagle"). It alleviates stiff, weak ankles and shoulders by bringing a tremendous amount of energy and heat into the shoulders, hips, thighs, calves, and ankles. This pose requires balance, which is never achieved by holding. Instead, be generous and allow energy to flow through your body, and balance will be the natural result. Hold each side for five to ten breaths. The regular practice of this pose prevents fat from being deposited in the thigh area. Let the eagle pose say no to cellulite!

#6 Tadasana (hands in namaste): *Tada* means "mountain"; *tadasana* means "mountain pose." Sometimes this pose is called *samasthiti*, which means "equal standing." From this pose all other asanas originate. Feel your two feet firmly and actively pressing into the floor. Touch the insides of the feet together, including the inner toes and inner heels. Reaching into the floor with your feet, draw energy into the body through the legs. Create extension through the spine by drawing the tailbone and pubic bone toward each other, allowing them to meet mutually. As a result, the pelvis should not tip forward or backward, thus allowing the lumbar spine to lengthen. Let the upper arms spiral outward, causing more space in the upper chest and across the collarbones. The chin should be parallel to the floor. Stand for however many breaths it takes for you to feel comfortable and at ease. This is a grounding and centering pose.

#7: Adho Mukha Svanasan: The common name for this pose is downward-facing dog. Like the headstand, this is an inverted posture in which the head is lower than the heart. It is more easily accomplished for beginners than a headstand. The body is shaped like a triangle. Press both hands firmly on the floor and lift the energy out of the wrists and arms. Press feet into the floor, lifting quadriceps strongly up. The feet should be hip-width apart and parallel. Drop the head and draw the chin toward the chest, gazing in the direction of the navel. This pose warms the whole body while it elongates and extends the spine. The knees receive circulation due to the lifting of the thighs. If you feel tired, this is the pose for you. It invigorates the whole system, leaving you feeling refreshed.

#8 Namaste (variation with hands behind back): Roll shoulders back and press the palms of the hands together, starting at the back of the waist. Move the prayer position up the spine until the hands are resting between the shoulder blades. Hold for five to ten slow, deep, full breaths. This pose relieves stiffness in the wrists as well as shoulders and corrects dropping shoulders and a sunken chest. Deep breathing becomes easier through regular practice of this pose.

#9 Trikonasana (triangle pose): Turn one leg out and one leg in. Press both feet firmly into the floor while lifting the legs up away from the floor. The kneecaps should be aligned over the middle of each foot. Activate the quadricep muscles by pulling them up strongly—this will allow the knees to come into a safe position. Make sure you do not allow the inner arches of the feet to collapse; instead, lift them up. Draw the buttock bones toward each other across the back of the pelvis. Move the front floating ribs into the body, allowing the lower back to lengthen and broaden. Bend to the side of the turned out leg. Place one hand on the shin of the turned out leg and reach the other hand up and over, stretching in the opposite direction to the turned in leg. This pose strengthens and tones the legs while opening the hips. It relieves lower back pain and reduces fat in the waist area. Hold steady and breathe five to twenty breaths.

SARAH BAN BREATHNACH

Author Sarah Ban Breathnach's **work celebrates quiet joys, simple pleasures, and everyday epiphanies.** The wisdom, warmth, compassion, and disarming candor of her number-one *New York Times* bestsellers, *Simple Abundance* and *Something More*, have made her a trusted voice to millions of women. *Simple Abundance* has been back to press fifty times and sold more than five million copies in the United States alone. Oprah Winfrey has called her books "life changing," and Deepak Chopra has named Ban Breathnach one of America's most fascinating women of power and influence.

Q I love the section in *Simple Abundance* about the relationship between our inner growth and our outer packaging. You refer to this concept as "spiritual beauty." What is the deeper definition of this idea?

Spiritual beauty has nothing to do with cosmetics or designer clothing, because spiritual beauty is repose of the soul. But our souls reflect repose only when we're authentic–being true to the women we really are. When I wrote *Simple Abundance*, I deliberately chose not to have my picture on the book because I wanted it to be each reader's personal journey. But as a result, millions of women started imagining what the living embodiment of "simple abundance" should look like. The two most familiar fantasies were Birkenstocks and granola or Laura Ashley's cottage sprig. But that's not me! I love sexy high-heeled shoes, red nail polish, hats and vintage clothing from the thirties, forties, and fifties–an era when women reveled in their glamour. But at first, this was a bit unnerving to some of my readers because it flew in the face of their expectations. This quandary brought up questions: What does "spirituality" mean? What does the spiritual life look like? Our society expects us to throw on sackcloth and ashes if we want to live "spiritually." Obviously, I disagree. Consider the ravishing beauty found in the natural world–flowers, animals, birds. To be spiritual is to be beautiful. One of the truths I learned on my Simple Abundance journey is that you cannot embark on a spiritual path within and not see it reflected on the outside. You simply cannot live a spiritual life and not glow.

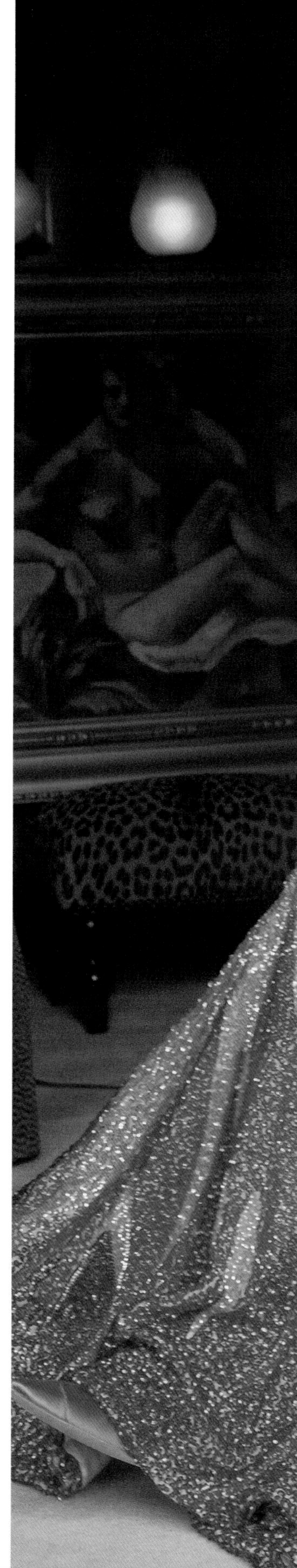

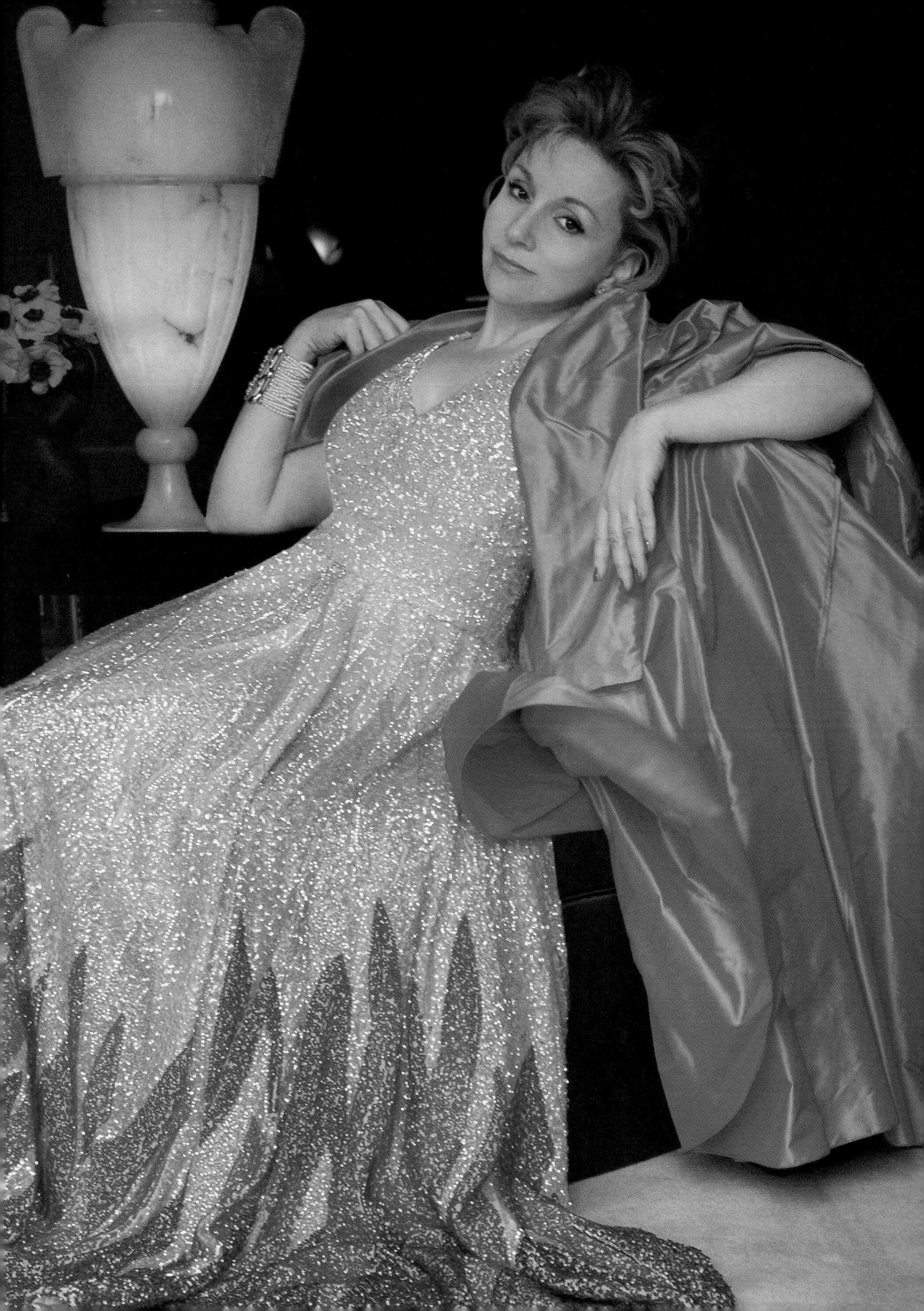

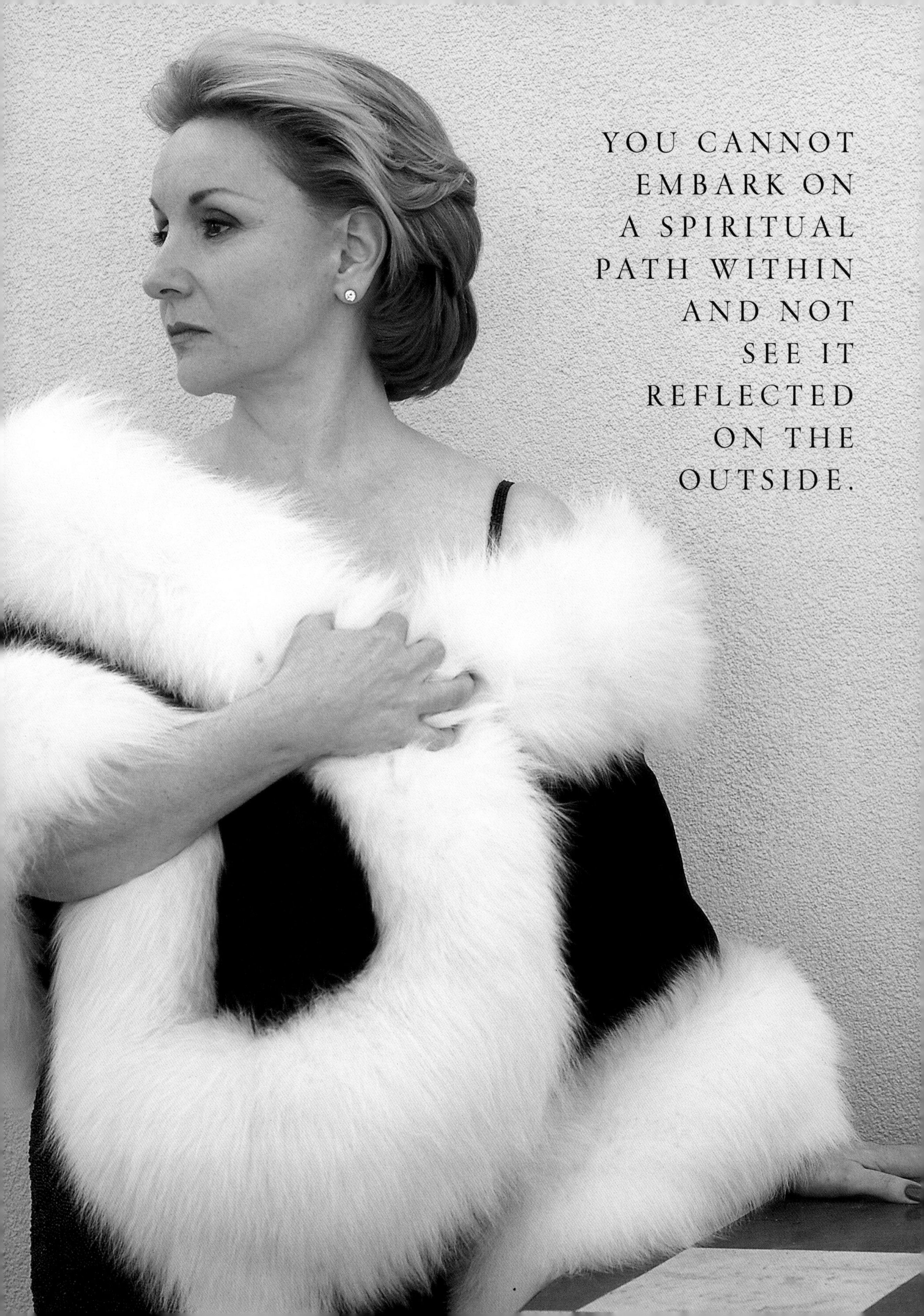
YOU CANNOT
EMBARK ON
A SPIRITUAL
PATH WITHIN
AND NOT
SEE IT
REFLECTED
ON THE
OUTSIDE.

Your **happiness** is not a frivolous luxury.

Gratitude is the most transformative force in
the cosmos because gratitude is love.

We are born in **passion** and we will die in passion.
Whether we live passionately is a choice we make with every beat of our heart.

The time, creative energy, and emotion you invest in
self-nurturance will produce priceless personal dividends.

Big **change** comes with small choices.

Truths to Live By

The more risks you take, the **luckier** you become.

Nothing hurts you more than your **expectations** of how "it" should be.

Our **relationships** with others are only as emotionally healthy, happy, holy,
and content as our relationships with ourselves.

The only wound the **soul** never recovers from is regret.

The most important promise you'll ever make and
keep is to love yourself into **Wholeness**.

TRUDY STYLER

Philanthropist Trudy Styler, with husband Sting, established the Rainforest Foundation in 1989 to defend the land rights of the world's indigenous peoples and conserve their environments. Today the foundation has programs in nineteen countries worldwide and offices in four. For the past decade, Styler has produced an annual benefit concert at Carnegie Hall, boasting the greatest icons in the music industry. Raising in the millions, the concert is listed in the *Guinness Book of World Records* as the single most successful environmental fundraising event in history. Styler has pulled it off while also bringing up four children, shuttling between homes in London and New York, acting as cochair and sponsor of the Human Rights Watch International Film Festival in London, and starting Xingu Films, a successful production company. She has deservedly been honored with the Center for Environmental Education Outstanding Woman Award, the United Nations Delegations Humanitarian Award, and the GQ International Environmental Award.

Q **How did you get started fundraising for the rainforest? And why has it become your cause of choice?**

It was by coincidence, actually. While Sting and I were on a trip to Brazil during the last leg of his concert tour, we were invited to spend four days in a rainforest nearly three times the size of Connecticut. While I was there I watched sixteen tribes living together in harmony with their environment. I saw pregnant women bathing their babies in the river and giving them the water to drink—not a sight that we're exposed to anymore. That was very profound.

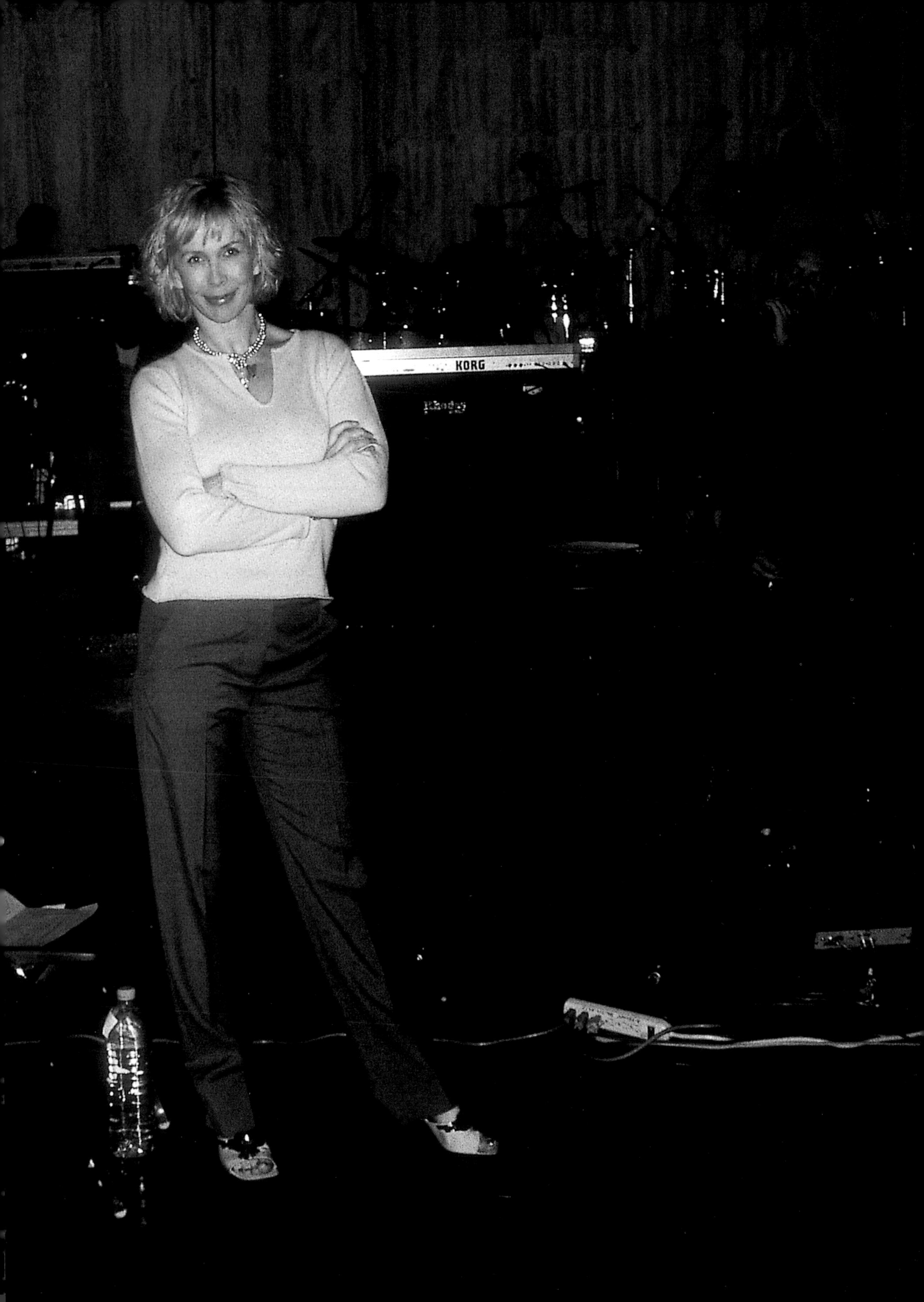
KORG

I then learned that the rainforests are being threatened by logging and mining. Vast areas are being burned and cut for development. We decided to try and save them. We met Chief Raoni of the Menkragnoti Kayapo, who beseeched us to help vocalize his people's plight in the heart of the Amazon rainforest. Using our celebrity we were able to spread the message around the world and share his vision of restored tranquility for his people. Through our efforts, and the efforts of everyone involved, we have made millions of people aware of the looming ecological and cultural disaster that faced not only the indigenous tribes, but also the planet.

It's alright for us to sit in our homes and think, "Oh, the rainforest is so far away," but when you see it, you realize that human beings live there. On a trip back to learn more about the Xingu rainforest, I nearly became the victim of one of those fires. I was flying in a twin-engine plane when an engine went out and we were being pulled into the fire. I thought, "What am I doing?" My normal reaction might have been to quit because it all seemed like too much. But in that moment I also thought if we get out of this situation it's because the work is so important. We did, but it left me scared and angry. What are we doing to our planet? What is all this destruction for—so someone can have a teak sideboard? We have to make the rainforest our responsibility.

Q How do you think that people who haven't witnessed these atrocities firsthand can develop a sense of compassion? How can we find within ourselves that sense of responsibility toward greater humanity and instill altruism in our children?

It's very hard for people to part with their money. I think that they really do have to become passionate about a cause in order to give time or money—it has to be in their faces. Everyone needs to revisit the virtues of charitable work; it's our duty as brothers and sisters to one another in this world. We need to impart in our children a sense of compassion.

Of course people will scoff at me and say that all of this is coming from one of the haves. But it wasn't always that way in my life. I grew up in a very poor urban atmosphere. I lived in government housing for a large part of my life, but no matter how poor we were, my mother always did charitable work, whether it was sweeping off the church steps or handing out needed rations. I believe in the laws of karma. It behooves us to give. It's not about having money or not having money. It has been my experience that in places like India it's always the poorest people who are willing to share their last crusts of bread with you and do it with a smile. We need to value what we have in order to appreciate what others do not. The positive side of this is that everything that you give away will return with interest!

Q I think this same dynamic is true if you want to fill your life with love or anything else. Give and you shall receive. Women seem to adapt really well to this philosophy.

Yes, I think that women are natural nurturers. We want to make things better; it's inherent in our personalities. More and more women are crusading for a healthier planet, whether it's about gun control or pesticide. However, we need to become more savvy to the laws of democracy and the role that politics play to reverse our loss of control over our environment, which in turn will directly affect the food we feed our children and the air that we breathe. As women we need to become more instrumental in change. Our voices need to be heard, and charitable work is an excellent beginning.

From the Heart

The development of compassion is truly the beginning of wisdom. It is also the beginning of greater spiritual growth. Anyone can give away money but without compassion it is impossible to give wholly from the heart.

Equality

It is through compassion that we recognize that all beings are equal, that we all have an innate desire to overcome suffering. When we acknowledge this ideal we begin to develop an affinity for all beings and are able to help others.

Give!

Giving is a flowing energy that not only helps others but also creates more for the person who is doing the giving. When you are selfish or frightened of generosity you stop the circulation. Giving and receiving are two sides of the same coin. Give back. Watch what happens!

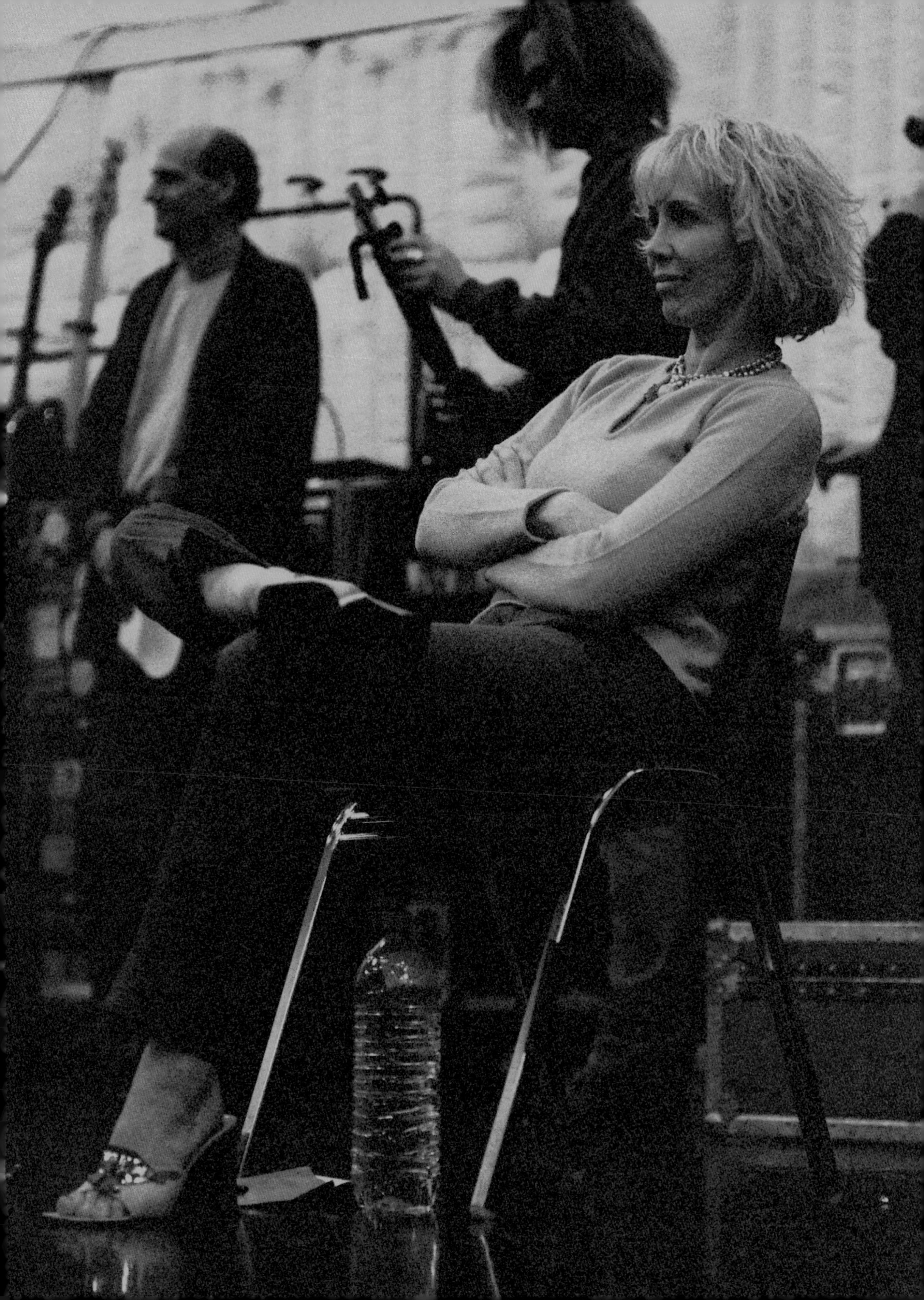

sweet CHARITY

Eight tips for more effective giving

For centuries, outstanding women have used their efforts and given their fortunes to bring about social change. The role of volunteer and giver is a traditional one for women, yet few people think of women as philanthropists. This is probably due to the fact that women don't give for the same political reasons as most men or expect the same recognition. There are also many economic, social, and psychological barriers to women's giving. Women own more than half the nation's investment wealth and in the coming decades can be expected to accumulate even greater wealth as they increase their earned income and inherit much of the predicted ten trillion dollars in intergenerational transfer of wealth. Yet until recently, few women understood their potential role as leaders capable of helping shape the future of society.

Many women are now striving to forge a path for others who wish to become involved. Women have made great strides in business, government, science, and sports; it's time for us to step up to the plate and enter the final frontier of the women's movement–philanthropy. The entire world will benefit.

Begin your philanthropy as early in life as possible. Even if you can't give as much as you'd like, your gifts will add up and begin to form your legacy.

Find your passion and focus your gifts rather than scattering them. Think about two or three areas or causes you want to support, and make this your philanthropic mission. Not only will your gifts have more impact, but you will find your giving more satisfying.

Work for parity in giving in your household. You and your spouse should have equal say about which causes your contributions support and the amount given.

If you can, give out of principle to the causes you are passionate about. Think of your philanthropy as you would a child–your investment in the future of our world.

If you don't have so much money, consider the strength of numbers. Organize with others to provide a pooled gift that can make a project possible.

Leverage your giving. Increase your impact by challenging others to support the causes you hold dear.

Have fun with your philanthropy. Celebrate your birthday with a philanthropic gift that you might not have thought was possible. Surprise your friends by giving in their names–or to a nonprofit of their choice. The possibilities are endless.

Spread the word. Teach the art of philanthropy to the next generation. Instill in your children, and the young people that you associate with, the values you treasure and your commitment to support them.

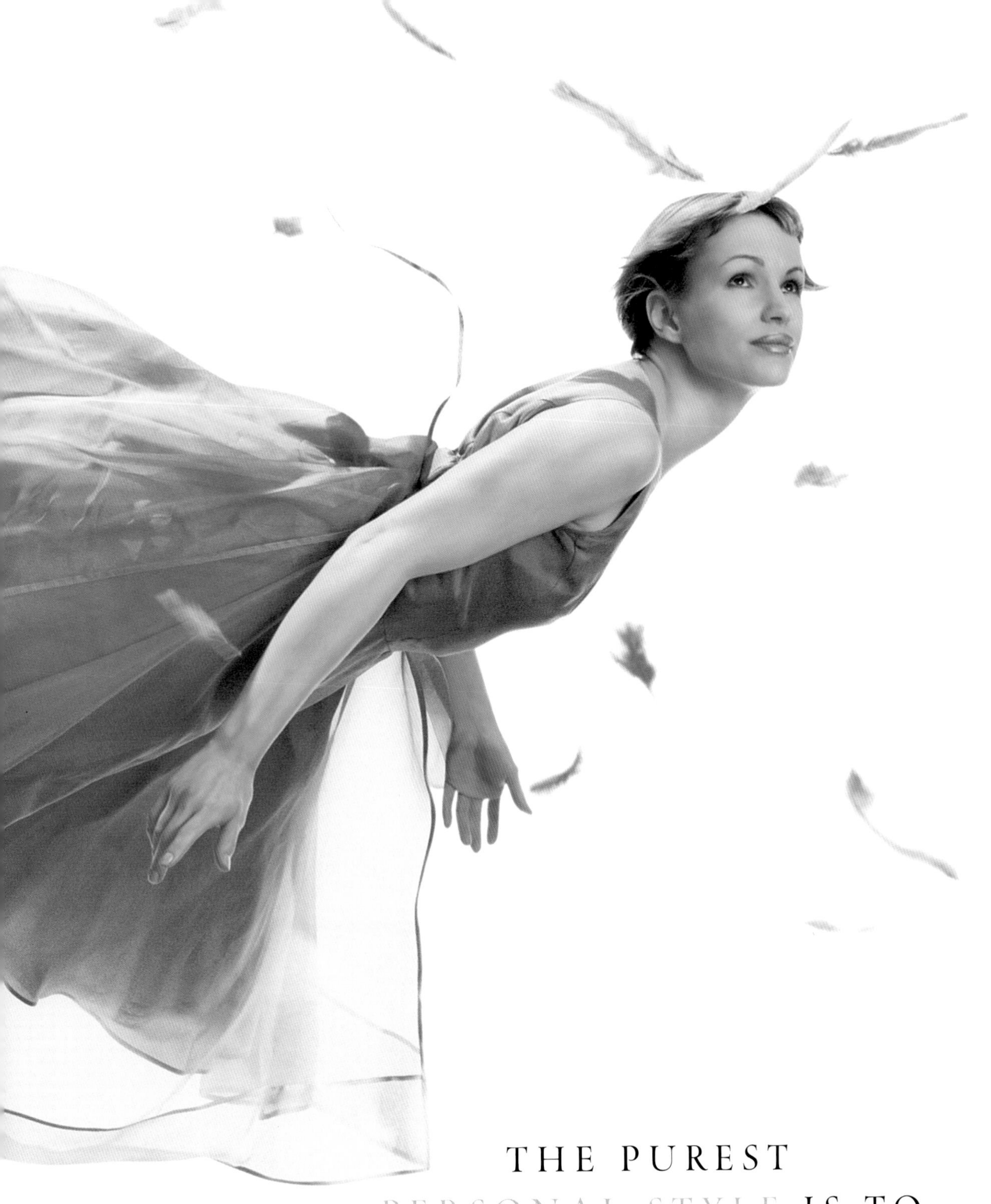

THE PUREST
PERSONAL STYLE IS TO
SEE BEAUTY IN
SIMPLICITY.

Q Marcia, how do you do it? Thirteen-hour days giving personal treatments and overseeing two spas in New York, one in Los Angeles, and a new place about to open in Miami. And you write the catalog and website copy to keep it entertaining. What keeps you going?

I used to believe that fear was my main motivation. When I was a child my parents didn't have a steady income. My father died of brain cancer when I was eleven. For two years he fought for his life. My mom worried constantly about money. I was scared because she never said, "Don't worry. Everything will be all right." She was going through her own suffering. So I worried constantly about starving or becoming homeless. There was no security. I was the mature child in my family even though I had two older sisters. I was the one who worked and studied hard. I felt responsible for everything. As I got older, I thought that the reason I was working so hard was to make sure I could survive. I never wanted to worry about having a place to live or being able to pay an electric bill.

I recently cemented an investment deal with a French company that wants to take Bliss to the next level. Now if I have a great idea, I can actually execute it without worrying, "Oh my God, will this make us go bankrupt?" On the other hand, I was really concerned that without fear I wouldn't have a reason to get up in the morning. I worried that once the deal went through, I would no longer be motivated or creative. But, thank God, I went into the office the day after everything was finalized and a reporter had called about a self-tanning lotion story. He wanted tips on application. I sat down and wrote the most hysterical ten points. I didn't have to worry about starving to death, yet I still came up with something funny. It was the biggest relief of my life.

Now I realize that what motivates me is my desire for women to feel accepted and comfortable with themselves. I hit puberty when my father was really sick. I was really young, grade four or five. I started to get hips and break out with acne. My skin looked terrible. I was a smart kid, but I wasn't pretty. Before my hormones kicked in I was hip enough to hang out with all of the pretty girls. But you know how teenage girls can be—whoever they decide isn't cool gets left out. Well, I was that person. I was tormented because of my bad skin. I was gaining weight, going through all of these changes so much earlier than everyone else, and at the same time my father was dying of brain cancer. Nobody helped me, and my mom wasn't exactly in the mode to get me to a dermatologist. She was drowning in the reality of my father's illness. I was drowning in insecurity. I was trying to support my mother and make her feel good. I was no longer accepted by my peers. My father was dying. I was nine years old.

I remember thinking, what is important here? My blemishes were so trivial compared to the other problems in my life. I learned to put my appearance in perspective, to laugh at my skin neurosis. I learned to use makeup and beauty treatments to make myself feel better—to bring out the best in myself. Beauty does affect how you feel about yourself, your confidence, and I learned that, especially when everything is going downhill, it can be the one thing that you use to make yourself feel just a little bit better, even if your skin is not perfect. It's that extra boost that keeps you going. Our goal at Bliss is to make people feel better, because we all know how it is to not feel good whether it's because of your appearance or feeling out of place. I try to make each customer feel special because maybe nobody else will that day. Regardless of the mood they came in with, we want them to leave thinking, "Wow, I feel great."

Q Your catalogs and website are peppered with funny quotes. Who hasn't over-plucked, permed too tightly, or self-tanned their palms instead of their skin? Why is humor so important to beauty?

For me beauty is all about having a sense of humor. I know how bad it feels to think you are unattractive, to have a poor self-image. I also know how good it feels to laugh at your flaws, let

Get Sleep

It helps your attitude, reduces the bags under your eyes, and relieves your coworkers. After eight good hours, you'll look prettier not only to yourself, but to those who have to deal with you every day.

Exfoliate, Exfoliate, Exfoliate

Why carry around excess baggage? Life is enough of a challenge without two extra pounds of dead cells weighing heavily on your T-zone.

A Glass of Wine

A glass of wine now and then improves your mood and reduces the wrinkles forming between your eyebrows. (Not to mention the benefits of potent grapeseed extract.)

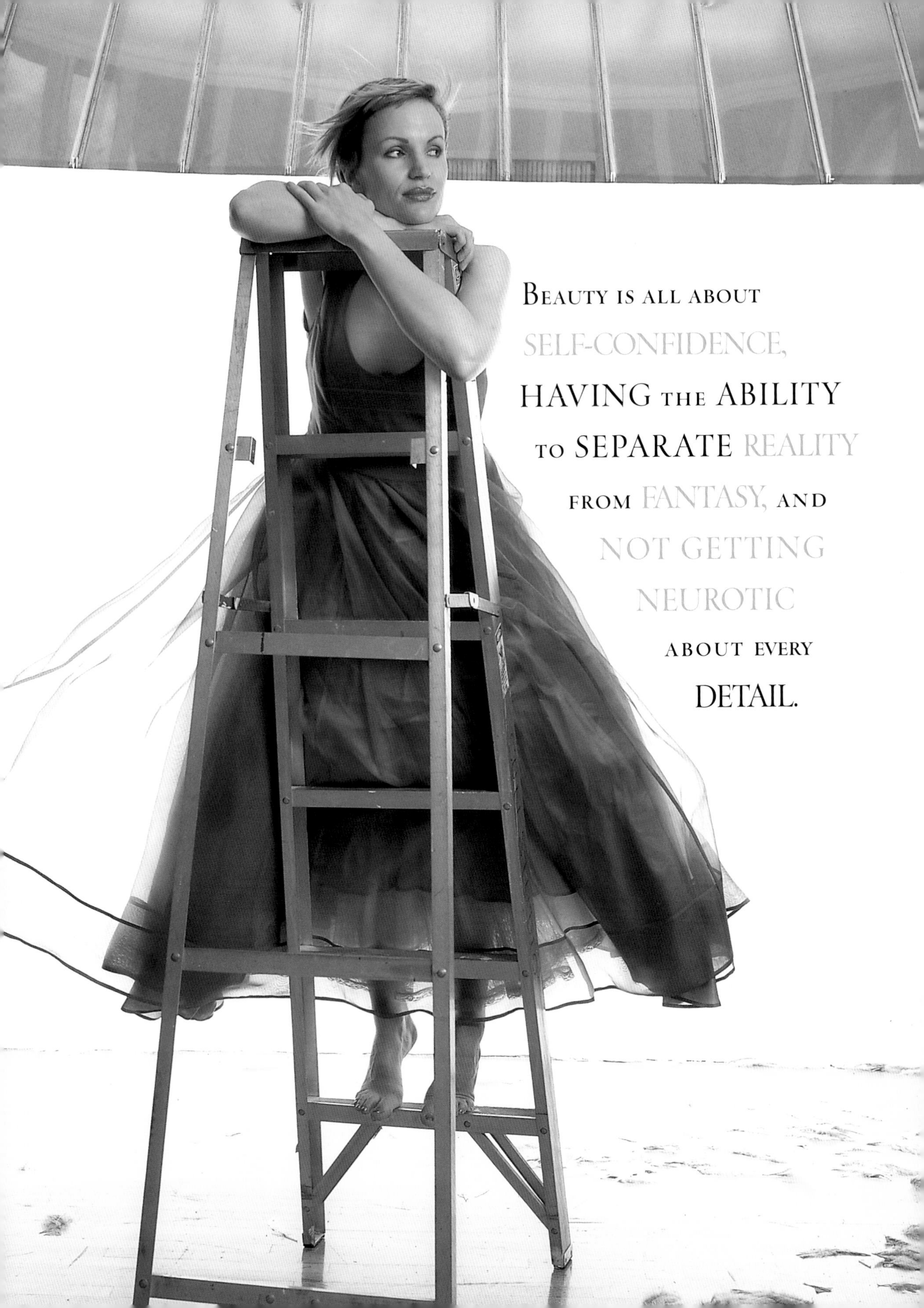
BEAUTY IS ALL ABOUT
SELF-CONFIDENCE,
HAVING THE ABILITY
TO SEPARATE REALITY
FROM FANTASY, AND
NOT GETTING
NEUROTIC
ABOUT EVERY
DETAIL.

go of that neurosis, and focus instead on what is beautiful about you and enhance those qualities. Bliss is about creating that positive, fun attitude even for people who can't come to the spa, but who are in need of rejuvenation, a laugh, or advice. We fill the catalog with at-home beauty tips and humorous lines like, "Hey, anyone in Lubbock need some lower body help?" and "Make cellulite think twice before settling down below!" Beauty is that little something special, not the be-all and end-all. Finding the hippest lipstick is not going to change your life or make you a better person. And I am always mindful that women look best when they are radiant with laughter. That's when they are the most beautiful.

Q We are bombarded with information and communication through the media, internet, cell phones, and e-mail. Women increasingly pressure themselves to know and do it all, and look good. What impact does this have on our appearance?

There is too much pressure to know everything. People stress about keeping up with it all, fearing that they'll fall behind or lose their job to someone more informed. It's insanity. And it's unrealistic. I try not to pay too much attention to what everybody else is doing because I find myself drawn into wanting to keep up with them. You can become paralyzed by competition when you should just be worried about keeping up with yourself. Set your own standards.

The great part of having a spa is that people need a break. They need to get away even for an hour and a half just to preserve their sanity—to step back and gain perspective. Lying down with no interfering communication is relaxing and rejuvenating. And if you can't make it to a spa, at-home treatments can be just as soothing. Turn off the phone, radio, and computer, light some candles, and lie down listening to comforting music. You'll feel more relaxed and able to be on top of your game. And rejuvenation is an essential ingredient to looking your best.

Q The vogue of fashion and beauty are constantly changing. It's a full-time job to keep up with it all. What advice do you give women who don't have the time or money to keep up with the pace?

There are many different types of beauty, and people should not worry so much about the images put forth by magazines and cosmetics companies, but realize that it's more about achieving individual beauty. Don't spend your time trying to look like someone else—spend it looking like yourself. I see so many women who come in every month, year in and year out, and it's always the same story: "What do you think of my hair? I just got it styled. My hairdresser says it's the latest look." Or "I went for a makeover and they gave me all the new colors to try, but I don't know if I like them." The person who spends that much time worrying about whether or not they have the latest look is always the least interesting to look at. Beauty is about self-confidence, finding your own style, and not getting neurotic about every detail. If you feel good on the inside, you look good on the outside. I see other women who get flattering haircuts, put on jeans and a ratty T-shirt, and they're smiling and laughing and having a good time. They exude confidence. They don't second-guess everything about themselves. Those women are beautiful.

Also, don't try to do everything. If you have terrible cheekbones, don't wear a lot of blush, or if you have terrible lips don't emphasize them with red lipstick. Pick your feature and really work it. Make it your signature style. Simplicity in beauty and life is the way of the future. Our lives are cluttered enough. Cutting out stuff makes it less complicated. We become free to focus on what is truly important. In my house, I'm all about throwing things out. If I haven't worn it in six months, it's out. Even though everything comes back into style, I find I still don't want it the second time around. I always realize I should have tossed it out the first time. People have an obsession with hoarding, but excess stuff clogs your mind. The purest personal style is recognizing the beauty in simplicity.

Stay in the Shade

Think three times before lying in the sun. It will save you tons of time in the mirror in later years—time that you would spend staring at the crevices on your face, wishing you'd resisted.

Don't Follow Fads

Don't get neurotic about the latest beauty fads. Concentrate on healthy skin, a great haircut, and good shoes. If your shoes are good, no one will notice how bad the rest of you turned out that day.

Quit Smoking

Really try hard to kick this habit. Smoking robs your skin of oxygen and diminishes the glow you're supposed to have. After that, there's no pretending.

GINGER FOOT BATH Soaking in ginger and cucumber is a detoxifying treat for your feet. It will help debloat your tired tootsies. Place warm water in a bowl and add shredded ginger and sliced cucumber. Adding some oil will help soften soles. Our favorite for feet is peppermint because of its cooling properties.

MILK ALMOND HAND SOAK
This soak is a great pre-manicure prep. After gently pushing the cuticles back with an orange stick, soak hands in equal parts milk and almond oil. The lactic acid exfoliates while deeply moisturizing. Sprinkle rose petals in the mixture. Rose water is a great skin clarifier.

CARROT SALT OIL BODY SCRUB
This strategic combination is exfoliating and rejuvenating. Try this at home or with a friend. In a bowl, create a paste of coarse salt, shredded carrot, and olive oil. You can also add an essential oil; choose one to soothe what ails you. Apply the scrub to your body in a circular motion.

CUCUMBER-PAPAYA FACE MASK
Cucumber is a great eye de-puffer and a veritable olfactory garden. Papaya contains papain, an exfoliating and purifying enzyme that's great for skin texture and pores. After a hot shower, place sliced cucumber on eyes and thinly sliced papaya around face. Leave on for 10 minutes.

DO-IT-YOURSELF TIPS

I THINK WOMEN LOOK THE BEST WHEN THERE'S HUMOR. THEY ARE MOST BEAUTIFUL WHEN THEY ARE RADIANT WITH LAUGHTER.

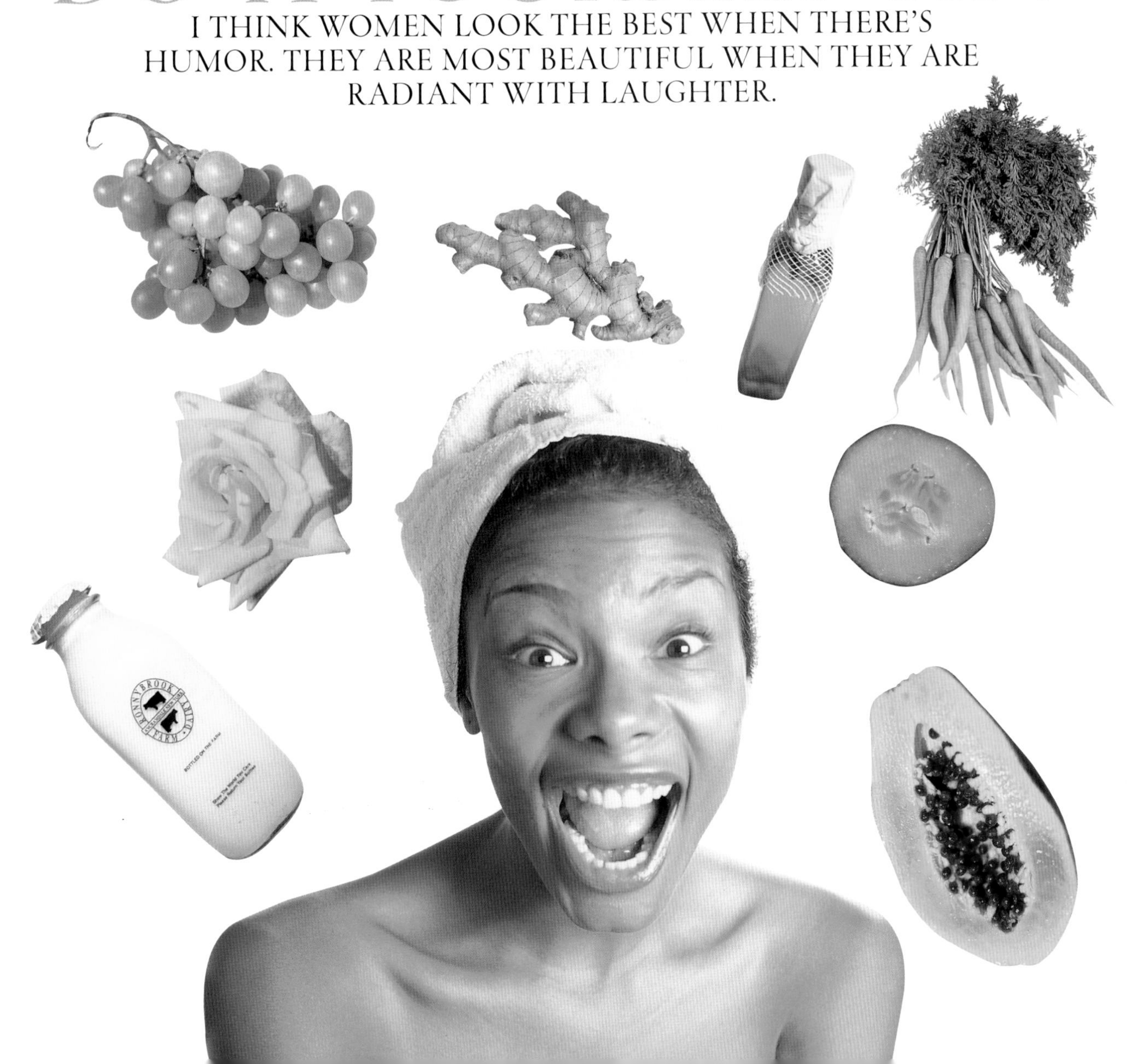

DONNA KARAN

"In 1985, when I started
Donna Karan New York,
I set out to design modern clothes
for modern people. . . .
Today that is still my mission.
I'm inspired by the artist that lies in all of us.
A sense of character. Individuality. Creativity.
The soul that learns from the past.
The spirit that anticipates the future.
The body that is alive with sensuality.
And the heart that knows no bounds.
That's why for me, expression lies in simplicity.
Why black forms the perfect canvas.
And a tactile caress has such sensual power.
Design must be flexible—a chameleon, an exploration.
Because modern souls don't stand still.
They keep moving forward, evolving, creating.
Forever inspired by life."

Donna Karan

Q **As I understand it, a pivotal moment for you as a designer was in 1974, at exactly the same time as another monumental event in your life, the birth of your daughter, Gabby, right?**

Yes. I was at Anne Klein, where I had already been working on and off for about six years. I was pregnant and went into labor at work, right there at the Anne Klein offices. The baby was ten days late, and the pressure was on for the fall preview collection. This was in the days when they still showed what was known back then as "capsule collections." Basically, Anne and I did everything, period. But she was in the hospital. And when I also went to the hospital to give birth, there was nobody to finish the collection. She had cancer. In those days, nobody knew you had it, or talked about it. It was not discussed. The office kept calling to ask when I was coming back. I remember needing to say, "Would you like to know whether I had a boy or a girl?" Anyway, I asked the doctor about going back to work, and he said, "What about the stitches?" I replied, "Don't worry about the stitches. There are plenty of seamstresses in the office."

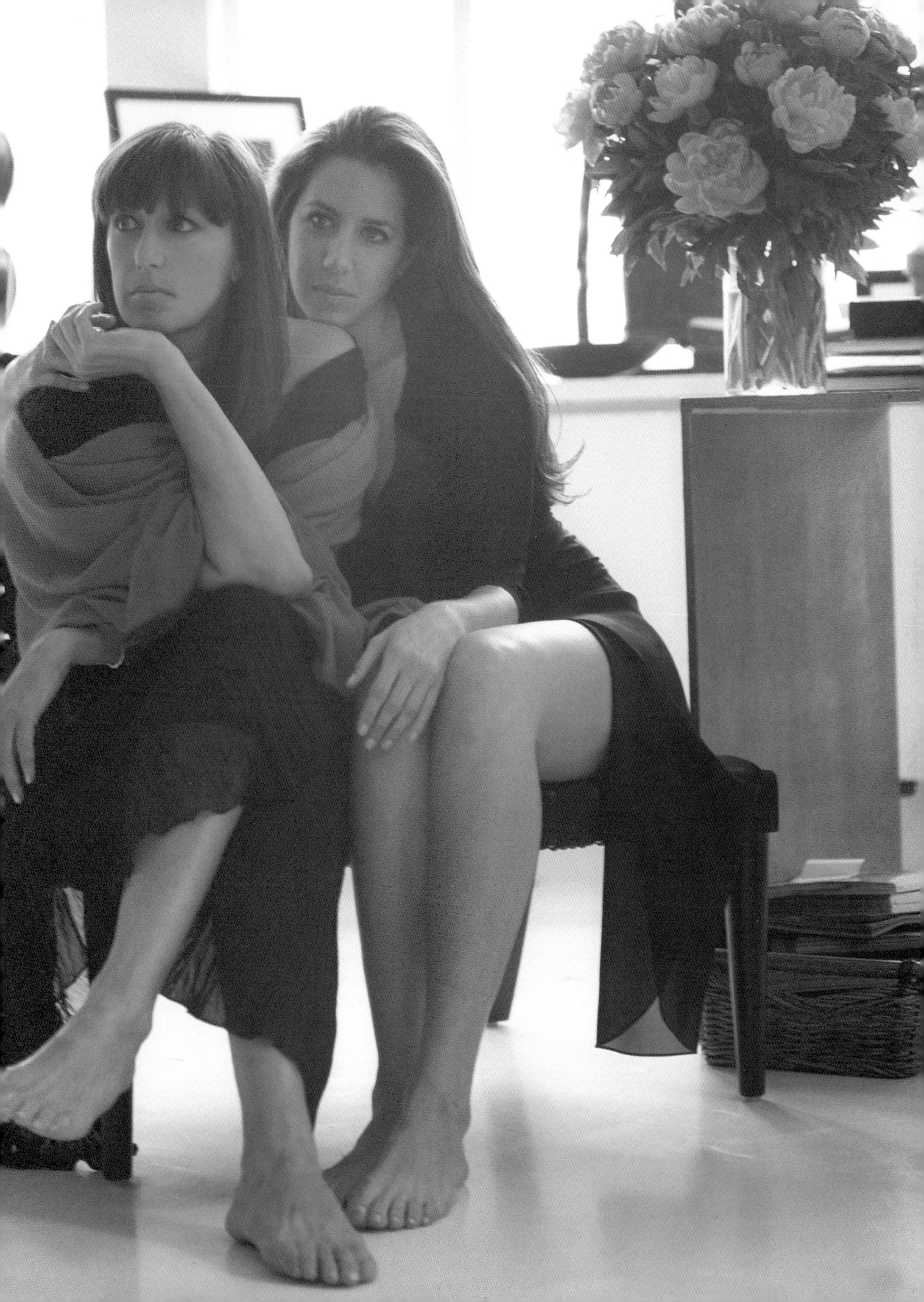

Q He must have known there was no stopping that situation.

Well, what he did offer is that I could return to work in a week. So, I went home, to a brand-new house in Long Island. There wasn't a stick of furniture, but we wanted to have the reception for the baby at home. So, here we are in the new house on Long Island, with a new baby. The table's made, the lox and the bagels are out, the guests are on their way, and the next thing that happens is that trucks are pulling up to the driveway. And then racks with clothes and half-made clothes come pouring into the house. Next, everybody from the office comes inside the house, and they're even bringing the dummies and the fitting models with them. The phone rings. Somebody answers it. We're told that Anne Klein has died. I felt very alone. I called up her husband, and he said, "Anne would have liked you to finish the collection. I know her, and that's what she would have wanted."

Q And you were instantly named as her successor. After a while, your friend from Parsons, Louis Dell'Olio, joined you as designer, but what a way to have it all fall on your shoulders.

Yes. I didn't even know what hit me. Anne was gone. I had just had the baby. And right before that, I had told them that I wasn't going to continue working. I had planned to stay home and be a mother. It wasn't that I didn't want to be a designer. I just wanted the experience of being home with my child. I grew up with a working mother. And it's tough. Talk about what you resist, persists!

Q You really kept Anne Klein on the map, and hauled in plenty of awards for it! By the time you launched your own company, Donna Karan New York, with your husband, Stephan Weiss in 1985, you were already a legend. How did you know it was the perfect time to leave Anne Klein and start Donna Karan?

You have to know when something is ready to be born. If you try to do everything within the same entity, it doesn't work. What I wanted to do was design clothes for my friends and for myself. I wanted to make a little collection that was all about need and desire. Being a designer led me to the questions in life that I constantly have—the questions that I have to explore. What do I need? What do I desire? What do I hope for? Originally, I wanted simple, comfort clothes, such as a few black pieces, for me and my friends.

When I say "my friends," I mean it literally and metaphorically. I mean women who, like myself, live a hectic life, who are in touch with their own sensuality, who know their own bodies, who know what they want. I was frustrated by what I saw was mostly available to women.

Q It sounds like a simple thing, but in fact, clothes that were actually sensitive to what women truly felt—instead of mostly being about what people thought women should wear—were practically revolutionary. Your idea started the way lots of new things start—with a dissatisfaction with what you were seeing around you.

It seemed like there was no bridge between sportswear and city wear. To me the woman was left out most of the time. The only American who had been exploring that territory was Halston. He'd had a modernity that was unique. He'd understood comfort clothes, and real ease, in a simple, sexy kind of way. Halston had expressed the possibilities of jersey. For me it was, and is, about cashmere.

I sensed that lots of women were frustrated. There weren't any options as far as I was concerned. I was looking for hosiery. I was looking for underwear. I was looking for a pair of shoes. I was looking for a bag, a belt. It wasn't just about the clothes. That's why I was so frustrated. I wanted a sense of feel and touch. I wanted to create direct contact between myself and the consumer. That was my dream: I wanted to talk to women—woman to woman. That evolved to wanting to talk directly to men, too. Men haven't been taken into consideration any more than women have been. For the most part, the whole issue of men's clothes has been reduced to either two buttons, or three buttons, or four buttons. Why can't a man wear his clothes separately the way a woman does? Why does it have to be about his suits, and then his sportswear? With men, first you go to the suit department, then you go to the sweater department, then you go to the shirts, you know, the system. Why does it have to be this way?

Q The thing that was said almost immediately about you was how much you understood women emotionally.

Hey, I live the same tortured life that every other woman does when I look in the mirror. What woman does not stand in front of that mirror and say, "I gotta go here. What am I going to wear? Look at my body!" I don't care whether she's skinny, or whether her ankles are this or her knees are that, one's confrontation with oneself is difficult.

We're all human beings. And I don't want to pretend to be something that I'm not. I think that's something that people have gravitated to, and can identify with. People want to feel good. Growing up I resented the looks that were imposed on people. I was allowed girlie-girlie stuff. And I wanted very simple clothes—even then it was black clothes and sweaters.

I never wanted the company to simply be called Donna Karan. I was sitting in my kitchen when I saw this Maud Frizon shoe box. It says Maud Fizon Paris–New York. I say, "That's it!" Then people started asking, "Well, what about the folks in California?" And we told them, "Everyone wants a piece of New York. New York is the hub. New York is international."

Q You seem to always be working toward a larger vision of what fashion could be in people's lives.

Well, our vision was very clear from the very beginning. It was never exclusively about clothes; we never wanted it to be simply about fashion. It was always meant to be about everything that touches a person's senses, starting with the sense of touch. For example, I had a mission to take ties off men. And why can't a woman go out in a T-shirt? The bodysuit that I did is basically a T-shirt. It was about giving women back their bodies and giving them back the comfort of their bodies.

Q Now you want to combine the market with the soul. Some say designers shouldn't think this way.

To me, if the artist's hand is lost, you might as well throw away the key. The minute it becomes bottom line, you're no longer in it. I don't think I could survive as a designer today if I didn't think this way. It's my water; it's my breath; it's my air; it's my essence. It's about what I react to, what inspires

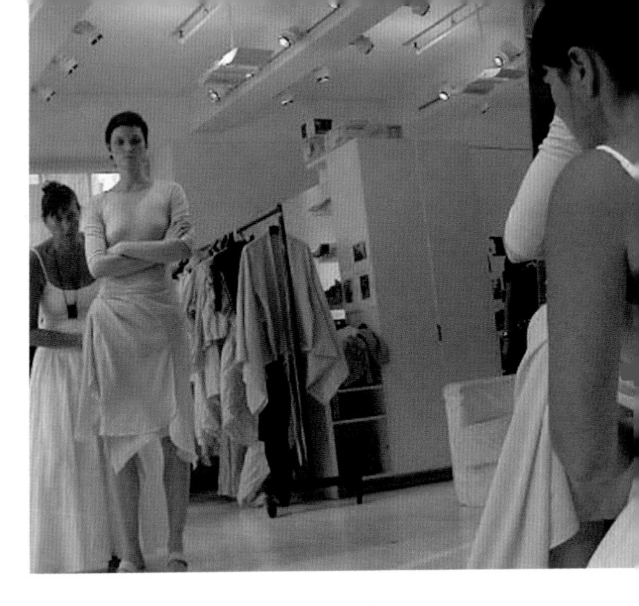

me, what my emotion is. For me, fashion is about touch, and feel, and emotion. And it should heighten your senses on every level. For Spring/Summer 1998, I was obsessed with creating the light of the bay that I had been experiencing. I would look at the rocks, and look at the bay, the light, the glass, the light in the sky, and ask, HOW do I communicate that sky color, that water color, that glass color? You have to understand why something means something to you.

Q And when you have to go out and buy clothes?

Forget it. That's why I became a designer! I couldn't stand it! In department stores? I hated the experience. It was so painful! I hated shopping. Going into a dressing room for me was like the kiss of death. And I know a lot of people have this problem. So, today, I want to create places where people get what they want. I don't want to confuse them. I want a woman or man to be able to walk into one of my environments and feel taken care of. I want them to walk in and communicate, and feel communicated with. I want to create that kind of retail environment—places that are compelling to go into. I'm going to do that more and more in the future—create places and things so that people can feel transformed, listened to, nurtured, taken care of, and special. There has to be something more to all this than just merchandise.

PERSONAL

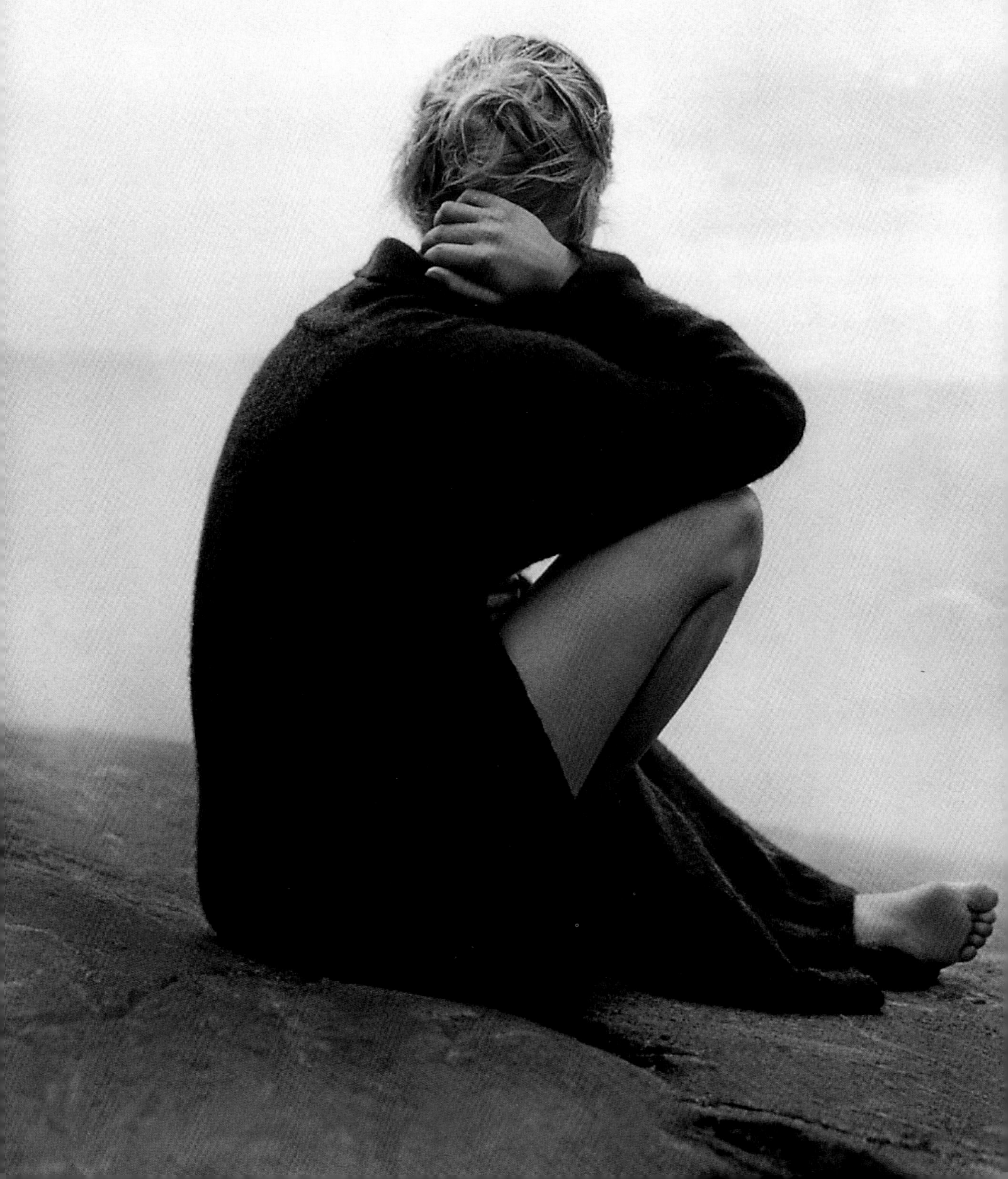

STYLE

Touch, Feel, Emotion

Find your personal style. Each woman is unique and beautiful. We each have a statement to make, a purpose, and a voice. We express them in our clothing choices, our complexity, our creativity. Express yourself. Be bold. Be honest. Look within and discover what fabrics, garments, and colors speak to you. Rid yourself of those pieces in your wardrobe that "just aren't you" and cherish those pieces in which you feel comfortable, confident, yourself.

Create clothing systems. I have always been an advocate of systems, especially when it comes to one's wardrobe. With just a few basic pieces creatively coordinated, you can move from mother to career woman to wife to athlete. The simplicity of having, and artfully combining, a minimal number of pieces keeps our lives uncomplicated while allowing us to have style, feel great about ourselves, and look stunning for every occasion. Once you master this art of paring down and being creative, it becomes effortless and beautiful.

Enliven your life with color. Grouping colors has always been a love of mine. I create whole collections with just one tone. The color speaks to me and I am inspired by it. Each new season, each new milestone in life has its own color, its own visual resonance. Notice the way different colors play off your skin, the joy you feel when you're wearing a bright hue or the calm of cool earth tones. Discover all the ways in which colors enrich your life.

Simplify. I have always found calm in simplicity. It is in nature, in the soul, in happiness, in peace. We let our lives get to a point where they feel out of control. Time is always of the essence; it never seems that we have enough to get everything done. Just a few steps toward making life simple can change it all. Simplicity gives us room to breathe. Release your life of clutter, of old, hasn't-been-worn-in-two-years clothing and makeup you wouldn't dream of putting on any longer. Let it go. Make a list of obligations, streamline your wardrobe, light a candle, and take a deep breath. Let the ease of simplicity work its way into the deepest parts of your life.

Relish your senses. Smell. Touch. Hear. See. Taste. Notice the deep feelings that well up when a familiar scent floats your way. Scents are intimately tied to our memories and can promote healing and peace. Touch has the power to relax, soothe, comfort; hence my deep love of cashmere, which continually caresses the skin. Sound moves us. The beat of a drum, the sound of waves crashing on a beach, a sweet song of love. Sound touches the emotions and brings us back with nature and our souls. Taste brings us pleasure and is strongly connected to nutrition and well-being. Take a moment to create an organic salad, treat yourself to a fantastic meal, or just enjoy the birth of spring with sweet red strawberries.

Relax. We are always going and doing. It is critical that we take some time out each and every day to do nothing. Take a bath, a deep breath, a walk. Feel the rejuvenation of these simple gifts you can give yourself. Clear your mind by meditating, get a massage, treat yourself to a pedicure. Empowered with the rejuvenating energy from moments of relaxation integrated into our lives, we can handle all of the demands that fill our lives.

Use your intuition. Women are blessed with the strength of their intuition. Find it, use it, relish it. Rely on those voices that speak to you subtly and powerfully. I found great inspiration in Laura Day's book, *Practical Intuition: How to Harness the Power of Your Instinct and Make It Work for You.* I have discovered that those hunches we are so often taught to ignore in lieu of reasoning and proof are really amazing tools that guide and shape our lives in phenomenal ways. Learning the difference between your intuition and emotional reactions takes practice, but to be in touch with your intuition is a gift that no woman should ignore.

Find time for yourself, alone. In these days of endless commitments, hectic schedules, and changing roles, women need more than ever to take time out to ground themselves and get in touch with their souls. Just a few moments out of the day can make all the difference. It is a time to refuel and rejuvenate. Breathe, meditate, visualize. Take a moment away from technology. Turn off the lights, light a candle, unplug the phone, turn off the computer, and shut your door. It can wait. Just for five minutes, enjoy yourself.

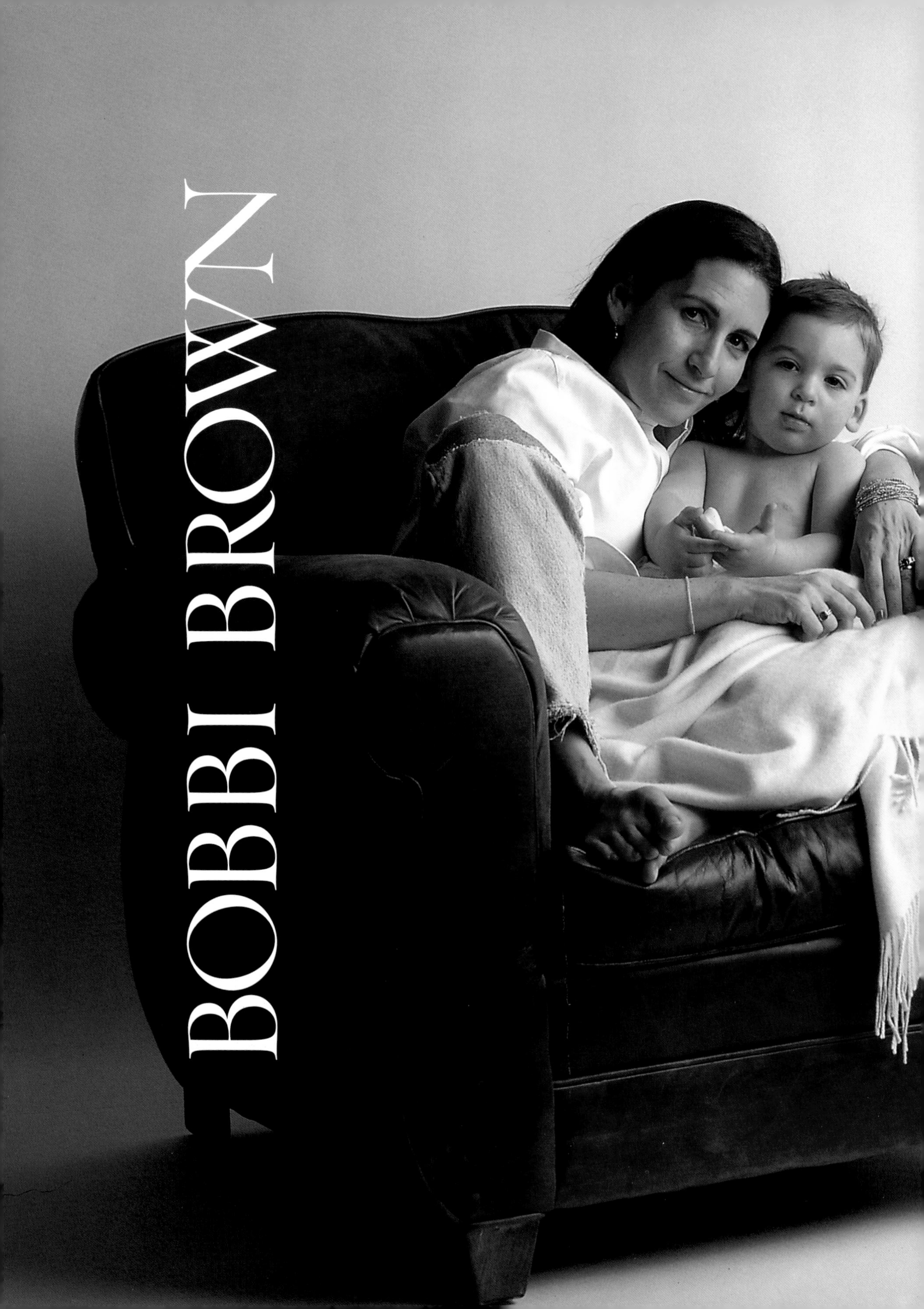

BOBBI BROWN

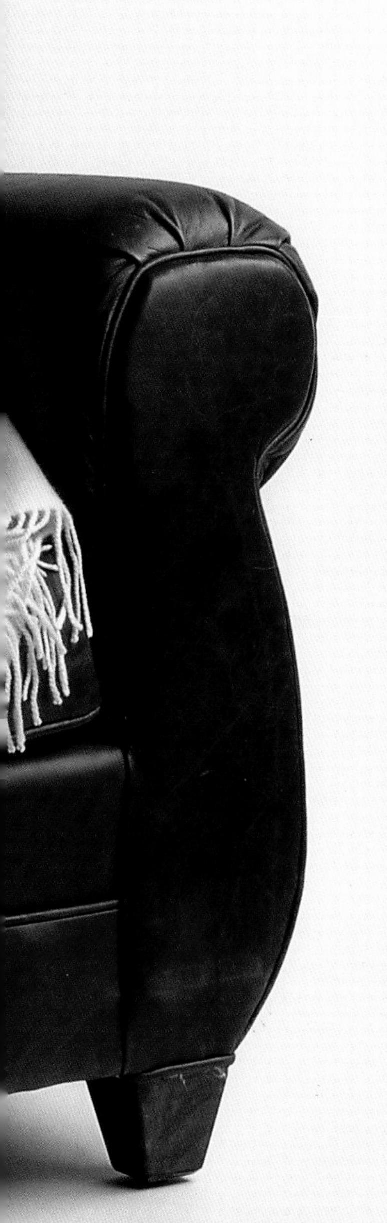

WOMEN TODAY
ARE VIBRANT AND
YOUTHFUL
LONG INTO LIFE.
THEIR INNER BEAUTY
AND CONFIDENCE
GO FAR BEYOND
LOOKING FLAWLESS.

When she was five years old, makeup artist Bobbi Brown raided her mother's cosmetic drawer and used a lipstick to paint the walls, the sink, and her face. Appropriately, she earned her theatrical makeup degree in 1977. She created Bobbi Brown Essentials in 1991, because she couldn't find lipstick that suited her natural style. Five years after it began as a stand with ten lipsticks at Bergdorf Goodman, the company grew into a multimillion-dollar cosmetics line. Still unfazed by fame and the fashion world, Bobbi says her idea of a good time is "being in the kitchen in big socks cooking soup with my three sons."

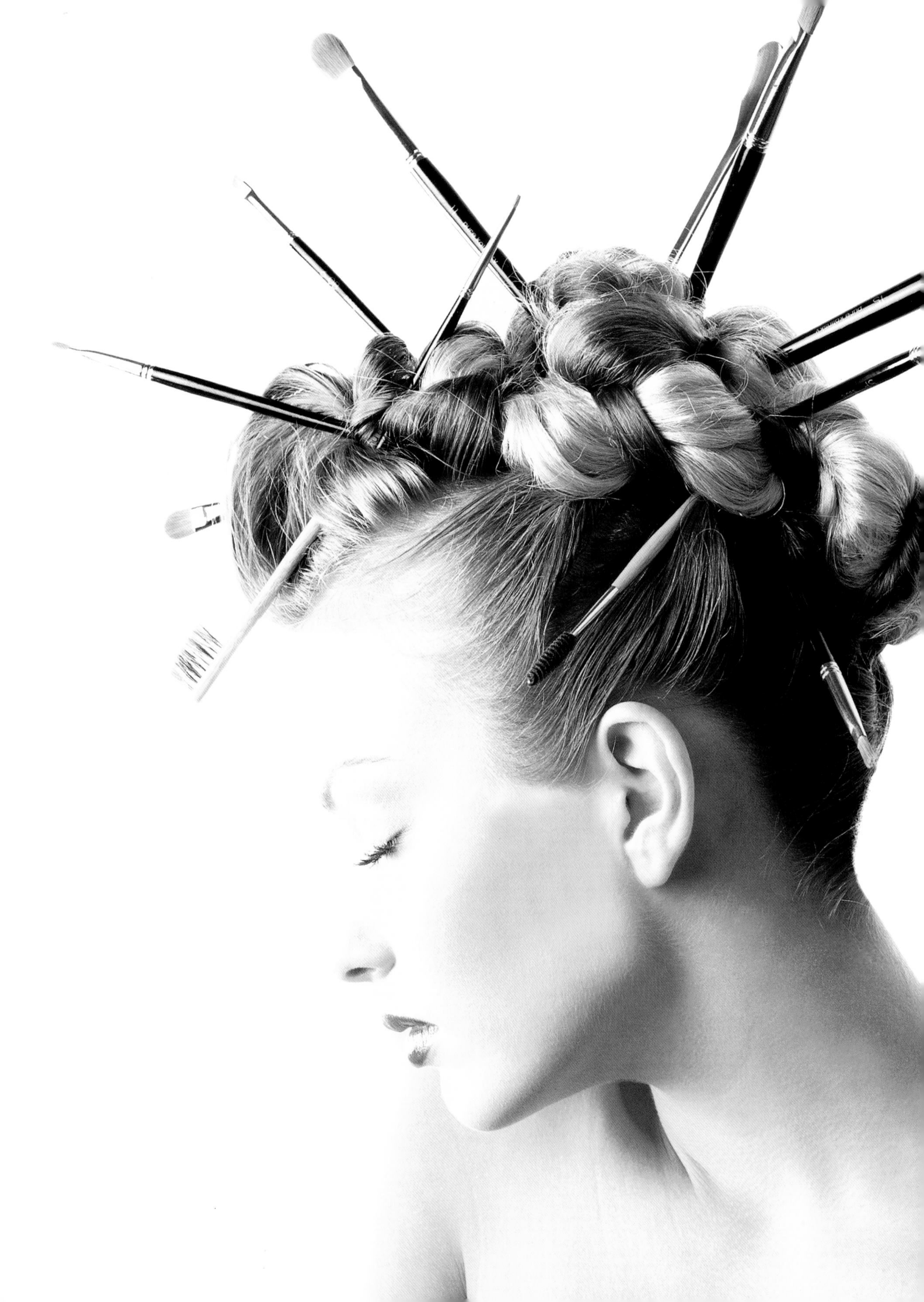

Q **Parental influence, good or bad, is at the heart of everything we do. I saw a photo of your mom in your book. She looked glamorous. Even though your style is very different, she must have been a big influence on you.**

My mother was the one who got me into makeup. She was really into beauty, glamour, and grooming. It was how I grew up. For me, the perfect night was staying home and doing facials, pedicures, and manicures with my mom, and eating a bowl of ice cream in my bathrobe. That was how I started.

Q **The fashion industry's standards are becoming less and less realistic for the woman who isn't a model. Yet your "keep it simple" approach to beauty seems to work for everyone.**

I think what's going on in the media is very unfair to women. There are some good things like the multicultural influence, plus-size beauties, and female sports icons. Those women are great. But then you turn on the TV and the girls are mostly teenagers who are too skinny or are altered to be perfect. It's . . . yuck! There are mixed messages out there.

Developing your own beauty style means prioritizing what means most to you and what makes you feel good and being realistic about who you choose to emulate. Choose someone who is close to your age and shape. Magazines that show real people can be useful beauty and style scanners. I have so many friends who are older than me—I'm forty-two—and they are so full of life. It's not like the women of my mother's generation who, once they hit fifty, were *old*. They believed they were old, they dressed old, and they acted old. So many women today are vibrant and youthful long into life. They inspire me with their individualism and confidence, which go beyond looking perfect and flawless. They are beautiful in their strength and inner beauty, which are brighter than any physical feature. It's timeless beauty.

Q **Beauty is a universal language between women. We are all interested in improving the way we look. Was it your own quest to be beautiful that propelled you into the cosmetics business?**

I try to look my best, as most women do. However, I wholeheartedly believe that no matter what kind of features you have or what kind of makeup you wear, confidence is always the most compelling element of beauty. More important to me than finding the right eye shadow or the perfect lipstick is striving to boost my self-confidence. I try to make a positive outlook my defining feature at home and at work—as a wife and mother, a makeup artist, and head of my own cosmetics company. I aim to make it the guiding principle of my life.

I think part of what drives me is that so many women are focused only on the negative aspects of their appearance. When I was younger I did the same thing. I was uncomfortable because I was not a cookie-cutter beauty. I looked nothing like Cheryl Tiegs, although my mother was always nice enough to tell me I was beautiful. The style of makeup I have created is a result of accepting who I am and using my God-given skin color, eye shape, lips—the whole package—and making the best of it. And that is the message I try to give to all women.

Q **I've heard you talk about "the here and now of beauty." So many of us suffer from the media pressure to achieve the impossible: to stop aging, stop changing. We lose interest in maintaining ourselves for our own satisfaction. We look at old photos and say, "Oh what's the point, I'll never look like that again."**

It's so true. My problem has been that I never thought I had achieved the ideal I was striving for. But when I look at old pictures I realize, for example, that my hair really *did* look great or I *was* thin. But at the time the pictures were taken I was probably thinking I was too heavy or that my hair looked bad. The problem is that we don't appreciate how we are at the moment. We're always aiming for some unattainable goal, even when we are fulfilling it at this very moment, even when we look great. So my motto is, accept where you are right now and be happy with that. Stop wishing you looked some other way or were younger. Allow yourself to grow and change and appreciate the process of maturing. Age brings its own beauty—the beauty of wisdom, experience, and confidence. Find the beauty in the changing you. Otherwise, it is so easy to get wrapped up in the media hype of "beauty is youth." Beauty is about looking as good as you can today. This idea should apply to your makeup as well. You should use makeup as a tool to feel your best no matter what state you are in. You should make choices based on your mood and look on a particular day. Then choosing what you need that day will become second nature, which is a whole lot more satisfying than following some unbending recipe.

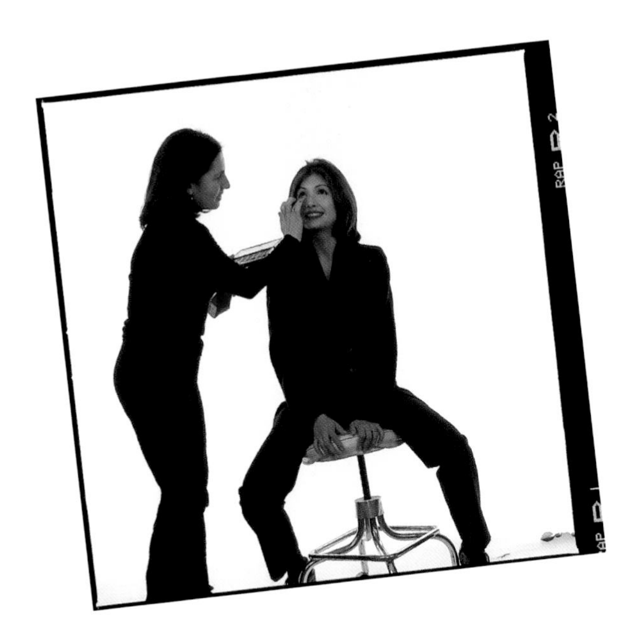

Beauty Through the Ages

Developing your own beauty style means prioritizing what matters most to you and what makes you feel good. For me, comfort is number one. Simplicity and practicality come next. Looking good comes third, which is very clear to me on the days I am driving into the city trying to put on my makeup at stop lights.

Many women become frustrated and overwhelmed with the world of beauty. Women of all ages desire to look their best, but some just don't know where to begin. This chart offers some solutions to the most basic problems for women in these age categories. Each tip offers a plan of action for moving forward with your looks.

70s

60s

50s

40s

30s

20s

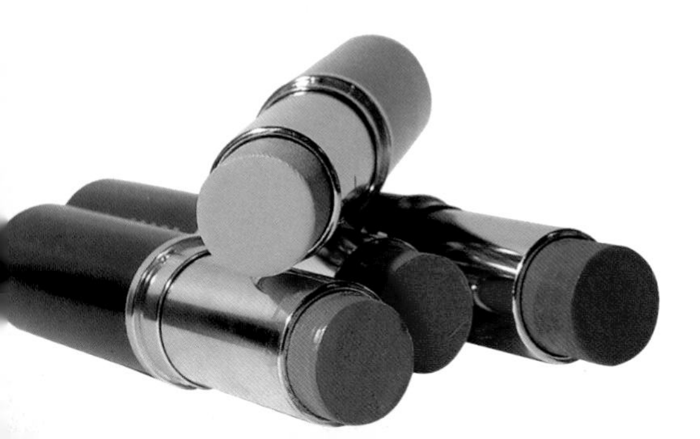

Energy, smiles, and happiness are often the miracle cosmetics for women in their seventies. More than ever, beauty at this time of your life is based on taking care of yourself. My strongest beauty tip for women in this age group is to moisturize. I have found that moisturizer equals youthfulness. Skin becomes drier with age, and products that are rich in emollient ingredients are crucial to keeping your skin hydrated. Make certain that your moisturizer is rich but absorbs completely into the skin so it can be worn underneath foundation.

As we get older we lose color on our faces and lips. It's important to wear a bit more color. Opt for softer shades that brighten your face. Blush is key as it provides an instant glow to the face. Cream blushes are a good choice. They leave a soft, dewy finish on the cheeks and are rich in emollient ingredients. Foundation is the surest way to get the skin that looks best. Foundation with a yellow tone looks better on almost everyone. (I can't stress this yellow tone foundation rule enough.)

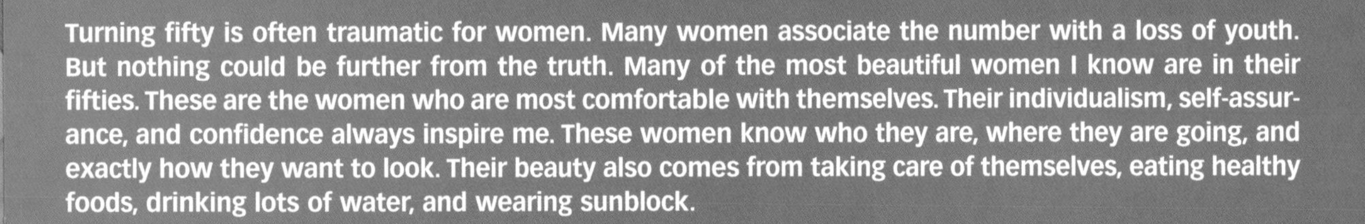

Turning fifty is often traumatic for women. Many women associate the number with a loss of youth. But nothing could be further from the truth. Many of the most beautiful women I know are in their fifties. These are the women who are most comfortable with themselves. Their individualism, self-assurance, and confidence always inspire me. These women know who they are, where they are going, and exactly how they want to look. Their beauty also comes from taking care of themselves, eating healthy foods, drinking lots of water, and wearing sunblock.

Age forty today is much younger than it was for your mother or grandmother. The forties now represent an age when women can be their strongest, sexiest, most vibrant, and most independent. Concealer is the one beauty item that really becomes crucial to incorporate into a woman's daily beauty routine. Dark circles under the eyes tend to become more defined in women over forty, and concealer can instantly brighten the face and lift a woman's mood. The right concealer is yellow-based (not white) and one to two shades lighter than your skin tone. Look for a creamy texture that is smooth to the touch. My trick with concealer is to layer it with a pale yellow powder to brighten this area and lock the concealer in place.

In your thirties you are still able to experiment with the trends, have fun with color, and be daring. You might want to try products that have shimmer textures and apply them to your cheeks, shoulders, or even lips. You can get away with it until your forties, when you will want to stick with a more classic look. In her thirties a woman will want to begin to pay more attention to foundation than she did in her twenties. Stick foundation is my favorite because it evens out the skin tone, especially in those areas that tend to be red or blotchy. Make concealer part of your daily routine. You will notice the difference in your appearance.

The twenties are the time to really experiment with your makeup and style. Pay attention to cleansing, SPF protection, and moisturization. If you start this early on it will become imbedded into your beauty routine. Even if you are only twenty, get into the habit of applying an eye cream. The skin under your eyes is so delicate; it's never too early to start protecting it.

NINA KELLY & ABBY HITCHCOCK

Acupuncturist Nina Kelly was born in Manhattan and raised in East Hampton. After graduating from Wellesley College, Nina entered the Worsley Institute of Classical Acupuncture (a five-element school) and also studied at the College of Traditional Acupuncture in England. In 1995 Nina began a practice in East Hampton, working with two fellow acupuncturists at East End Acupuncture Associates. After marrying another fellow acupuncturist, she opened a second practice in Soho. Nina is nationally certified and state licensed to practice acupuncture and specializes in acupuncture for facial rejuvenation.

Chef Abby Hitchcock graduated with a blue ribbon diploma from Peter Kump's New York Cooking School. She has worked at the Tea Box Cafe at Takashimaya, at Vong, and as an editor at BBC *Vegetarian Good Food Magazine.* She started a catering business with a unique approach to food combinations that has attracted such discriminating celebrity clients as Madonna and Christopher Reeve. Abby opened her own bistro, Camaje, in Greenwich Village two years ago and is currently in the process of opening her second New York restaurant.

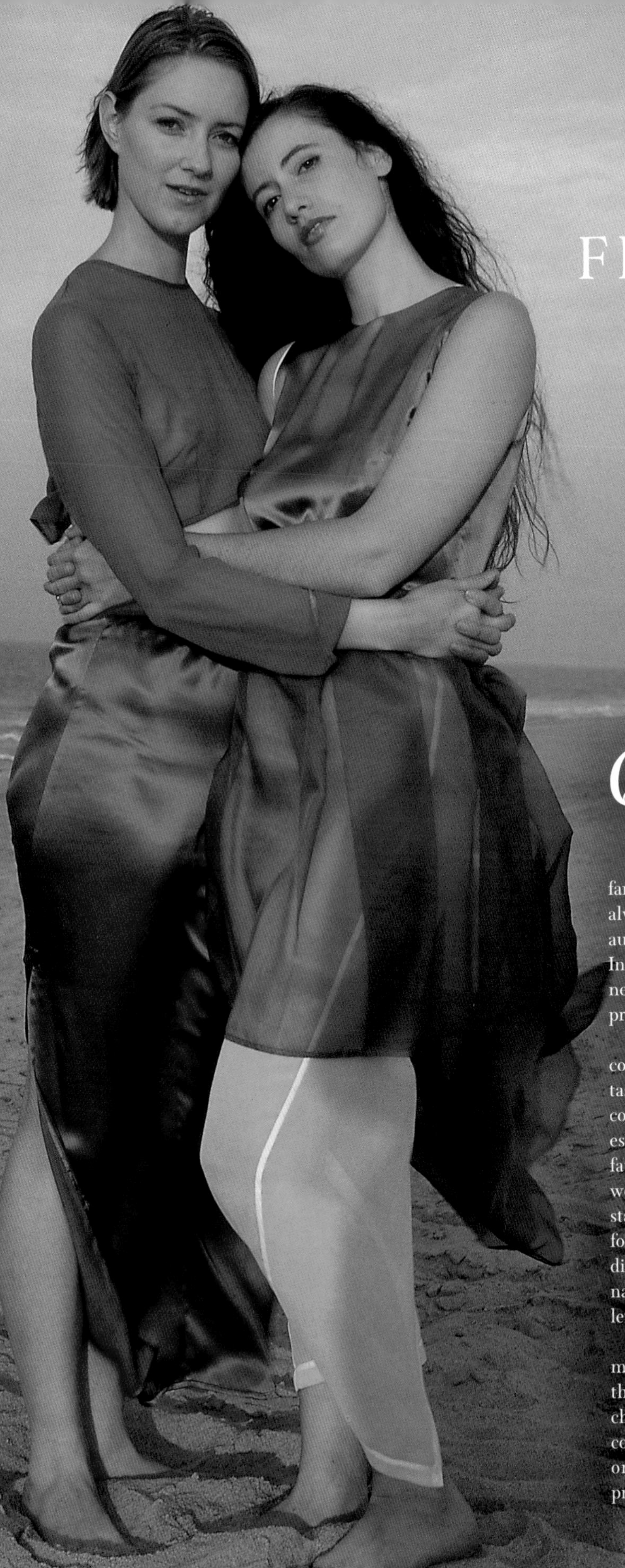

THE GROWTH OF TRUE FRIENDSHIP IS A LIFELONG AFFAIR.

Q How did you two end up in your current professions?

ABBY: My father loved cooking and creating fantastic meals out of international dishes. He was always trying new recipes. He taught me to use authentic ingredients; we used Indian spices for Indian food and shopped in Chinatown for Chinese food. He always emphasized the use of fresh produce and herbs. Most of it he grew himself.

I was quite mean to my mom about her cooking. I would tell her how horrible her food tasted compared to my dad's. But really, her cooking was not at all bad; it was just uninteresting because she was really cautious about the fat content. Many of her family members had weight problems, and her mother was constantly scolding them about eating fattening foods. Of course, the result was that they immediately wanted to eat everything that wasn't nailed down. Eating disorders were a real problem in her family.

Ultimately it was my father who persuaded me to go to culinary school. I had always thought that I would become a midwife and work with children. I didn't change my mind until I got to college, where I was always cooking for everyone, and realized I really didn't want to do premed.

Q **As a waitress in college I encountered a lot of very aggressive chefs in the kitchen—it seemed like such a macho thing. When it comes to the professional kitchen, women just seemed to get pushed out. And isn't that ironic? The kitchen is traditionally the woman's domain.**

ABBY: Yes, there are very few women in culinary school for this reason, and many of the women who do go don't end up in the kitchen. Instead they do magazine work or reviewing or styling. But people who are really serious and focused welcome women into the kitchen. I was fortunate; my first professional cooking experience, as an intern at the Tea Box in New York, was very positive. It was run by a woman named Ellen, who created a wonderful dynamic in the kitchen. But then I went to work in a stereotypical kitchen in London, where the men did the hot line and the women did pastry and salad. I was constantly saying, "No, I can do that," and they'd say, "Oh, are you sure you don't want me to get that, love?" All these side comments and sexual innuendoes. One guy never stopped talking to me about sex. Though he did make one nice comment to me. He said, "You could work here. We would hire you because you are obviously very committed." I wasn't sure what was going to make me happy.

Then an opportunity came up to work in TV on *Martha Stewart Living*. Then things started to happen. I met my partner, Patrick, and we started a restaurant called Camaje in New York. We keep it small and intimate, which allows us to offer fresh foods daily and imaginative menus. Now, as well as running my restaurant, I do private catering. It's very interesting because you see what people eat. Christopher Reeve is one of my catering clients. Eating is one of the only physical things he can really enjoy, but we keep his meals low fat because he can't burn off calories. I also work developing recipes for major manufacturers, like Sarah Lee and Uncle Ben's.

Stay in Touch with Close Friends

Friends make you feel at ease, happy, and able to be yourself. Keep a social network that can support and feed you. We all need human contact and, above all, love.

Combine Treatments

When you see an acupuncturist, you don't have to give up your physician or go off all your medications. Bridging between the different systems is key. Both allopathic and complementary forms of medicine have things to offer the patient.

Focus on Your Food

Make the meal an experience. Create a positive atmosphere with relaxing music, candlelight, and people you like. Atmosphere is something that the Chinese talk about in the study of feng shui. Make sure you are comfortable wherever it is you eat, that your couch or chair is comfortable, and that the lighting is not too harsh.

For me it's all about maintaining the idea that the breaking of the bread and the sharing of meals together mean more than the satisfaction of a need. There is a strength that occurs when we take the time to bathe in the comfort of our meals together.

Q **Nina, did your parents also influence your choice in career?**

NINA: I grew up in East Hampton, which was great, but my parents had their difficulties. My father had been a missionary. He likes to be in charge, so he has the perfect personality to go out into a developing area and do that kind of work. But it was hard for him to come back and do a typical American job, and he ended up skipping around to many different jobs. My mother supported us a lot of the time by baking bread. She went to the local water mill, which wasn't functional, and persuaded them to start milling. Then she bought a big stack of wheat and had them mill the wheat. It was amazing.

Q **Acupuncture has only recently gained popularity and been brought into public knowledge. What made you interested in such a cutting-edge field?**

NINA: I wanted to be a midwife. I read an article about water birthing when I was in high school and was amazed. And I was a good student so I thought I'd go to medical school. While in university I did my junior year abroad in France. That really changed things for me. I was looking to take a yoga class and ran across a qi gong class, which I knew nothing about. I learned that it is a martial art, but also a healing art. The instructor became a great influence on me. When I came back to this country, I had to decide if I wanted to go straight to medical school. I knew I wanted to practice an alternative and holistic type of medicine. And I really liked to work with my hands.

That's when I met Carol Sigler, an acupuncturist who's been practicing for twenty years or more. She inspired me to go to acupuncture school. I liked the idea of integrating the body, mind, and spirit. And acupuncture is a combination of art and science. There are very specific points that you have to hit,

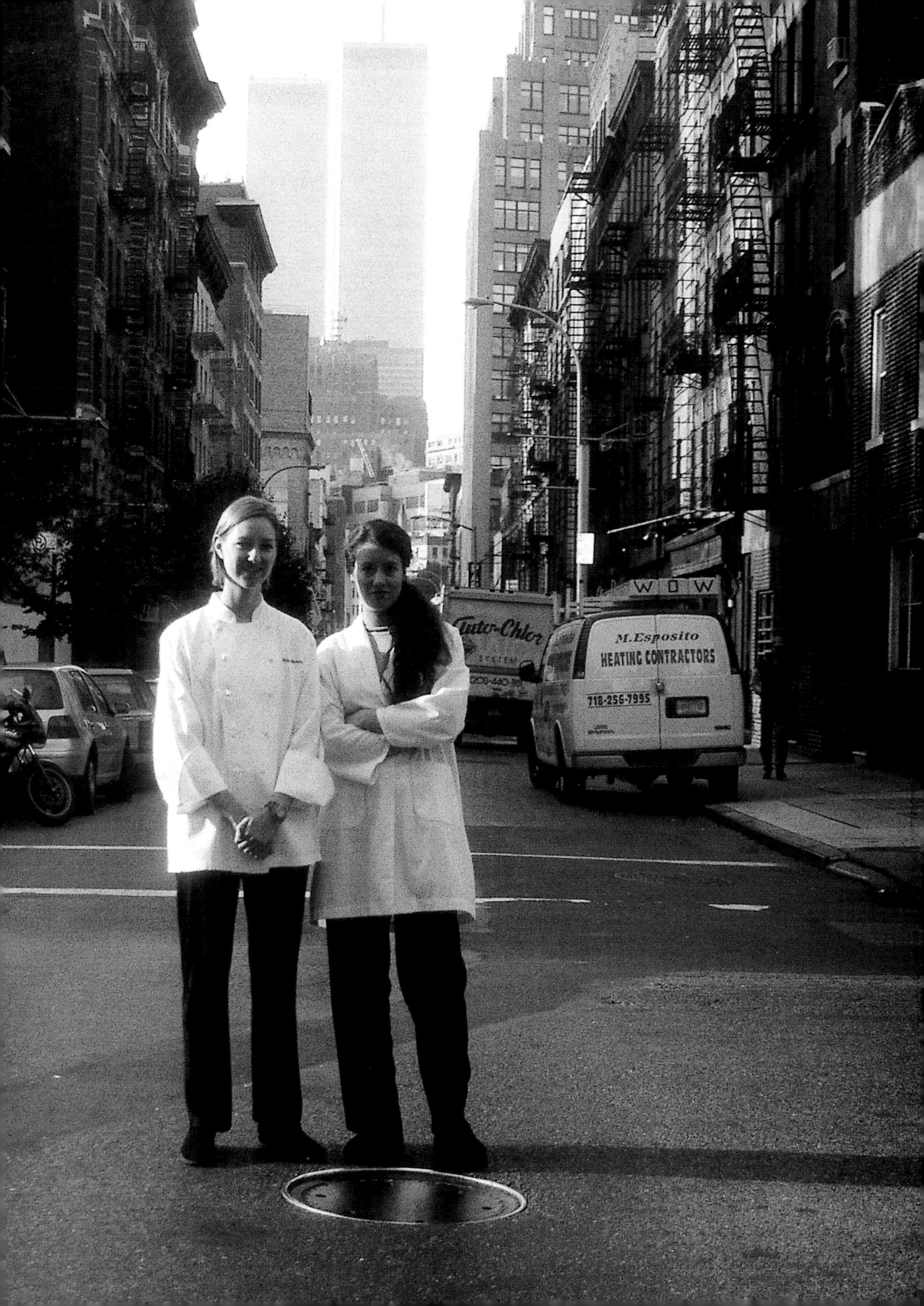
W O W
Auto-Chlor
M.Esposito
HEATING CONTRACTORS
718-256-7995

but there is an artistic way of using the points, of working with them to move the energy in the body. The root of five-element acupuncture is the belief that a person is a microcosm of the macrocosm, the universe. The laws that govern nature also govern the body. We don't talk about a sickness in terms of symptoms. We look at the color, sound, odor, and emotion of the patient. These are the golden keys. We notice the slight color that comes off the face, usually around the temples or mouth. We must be aware of the person's voice. For instance, they might sound angry, but maybe there's fear underneath the anger. We have to notice those subtleties.

How does the practice of acupuncture relate to women? My mother has been in and out of hospitals my whole life and I always thought she didn't get proper care because she was a woman, and all the diagnostic tests and statistics are based on men.

NINA: Most medical statistics are based on men, but acupuncture focuses on the individual. It's about listening to what each individual has to say and treating each person as a unique being with a unique energy makeup. Gender is not as much of an issue. Acupuncture is based very much on communication. Patients know I'm there to listen, but it can take some time for them to open up because they're not used to health care practitioners who listen. They have been taught to hide signs of pain, especially women. So I ask a lot of questions about medical history and body systems. The first session takes about two hours. A very important part of my job is teaching patients how to let me know what their true state is. This also helps them learn about their own bodies and to be clear about how they feel physically and emotionally.

I treat women for all types of physical and psychological pain. Oftentimes I relieve their pain right there on the table, but then they come back to me after a couple of weeks and report that they experience other benefits. Commonly, they sleep better and feel emotionally more grounded. I also do acupuncture for facial rejuvenation or acupuncture face-lifts for a lot of women. Usually a person requires a series of twelve treatments to get the maximum benefit. I have a patient in her early sixties who had had about six when she ran into a friend she hadn't seen in a while. The friend asked, "What have you done?" The patient said, "Oh, nothing. I just I eat well." The friend didn't believe her and asked if she'd gotten a mini face-lift. It took her a while until she admitted what she was doing. The difference was really that dramatic and she didn't even go through surgery.

I think it's very important to balance treatment between medical doctors and alternative health care givers such as massage therapists and acupuncturists. The preventive aspect of alternative medicine is so critical. We need to go to acupuncture or massage to continue to feel well rather than only seeing a doctor when we're sick. It's the same as changing the oil in a car to keep it running well. We need to eat well and get a massage every so often. In fact, Chinese medicine talks a lot about diet and balancing the yin and yang, or energy, of the foods we eat. Yin and yang is at the base of everything I do. I don't try to fix someone. I aim to balance their energy. A patient isn't going to be 100 percent well all of the time. It's okay to have the ups and downs, but I aim for them to be healthy overall. I counsel them away from extremes, toward balance.

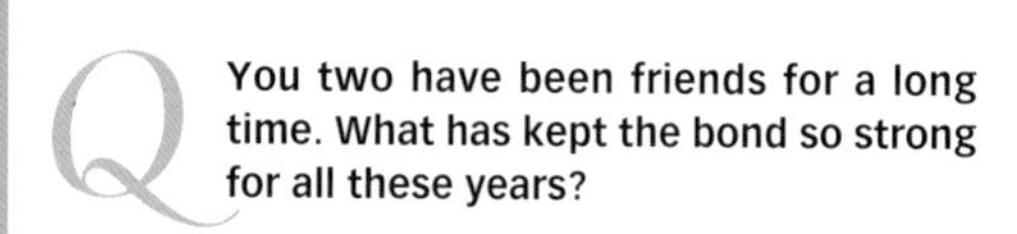

You two have been friends for a long time. What has kept the bond so strong for all these years?

NINA: Definitely food. Also, our professions are closely related. They are both health services. Eating well is as important to health as preventive medicine. And we both are concerned with educating people about how to stay in balance. We come from families of strong women and liberal backgrounds in which women are important. And we both went to women's colleges. That kind of experience provides a powerful example of the strength and community of women.

The Meal Plan

"Eat breakfast like a queen, lunch like a princess, and dinner like a pauper" to keep your stomach at its happiest. The Chinese clock says that different organ systems in the body have more energy (and thus work more efficiently) at specific times of the day.

AM or BM?

The Chinese clock also says that the large intestines have the most energy in the morning, between 5 and 7 A.M. Constipation is a common problem. Using the bathroom during these early hours regularly for a month can greatly improve this bodily function.

Cut Out the Coffee

Cut out or drastically reduce your intake of coffee. Coffee is something we CAN quit. There is a period of three days or so when you will feel a dull headache, but if you are determined, it is one of the easier substances to quit. If you feel you need some caffeine, drink green tea instead; it contains less caffeine in a much healthier form for the body to use.

YIN AND YANG
IS AT THE BASE OF EVERYTHING I DO.
I COUNSEL MY PATIENTS AWAY
FROM EXTREMES—TOWARD BALANCE

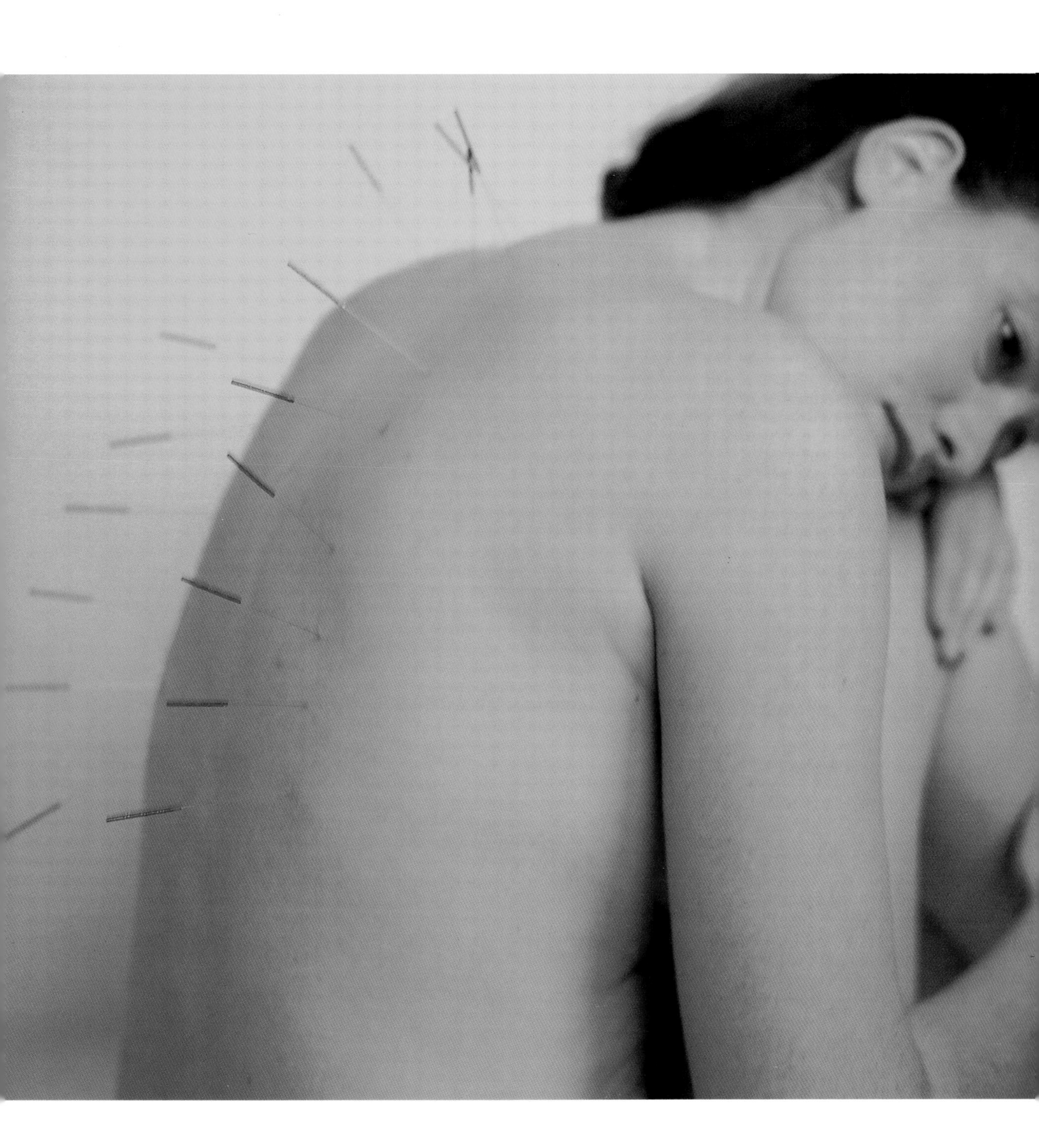

INTEGRATE

BODY, MIND, AND SPIRIT

Acupuncture is a combination of art and science. The laws that govern nature also govern the body.

HEAD

HEADACHES

There are many different kinds of headaches and ways to treat them. A lot of us have heard of the "headache point" located in the fleshy part between the thumb and the index finger on the back of the hand. This is a great point to stimulate for relieving frontal or sinus headaches. If the headache is between the eyebrows or on the side of the neck, rub the side of the hand by the pinky finger, either right where the pinky joins the hand or halfway down the carpal bone on the hand itself. For a headache that's on the temples or at the base of the back of the head, rub the knuckle between the ring and pinky fingers. This might be the best point for one-sided migraines or hormonal headaches. In all of these areas, press to find the most tender points and massage them firmly. If the pain is mostly on one side of the head, rub the opposite hand. If the pain does not subside within a few minutes of rubbing, try another tender point. Organic peppermint essential oil is great for headaches—put a drop on the temples and at the back of the base of the head.

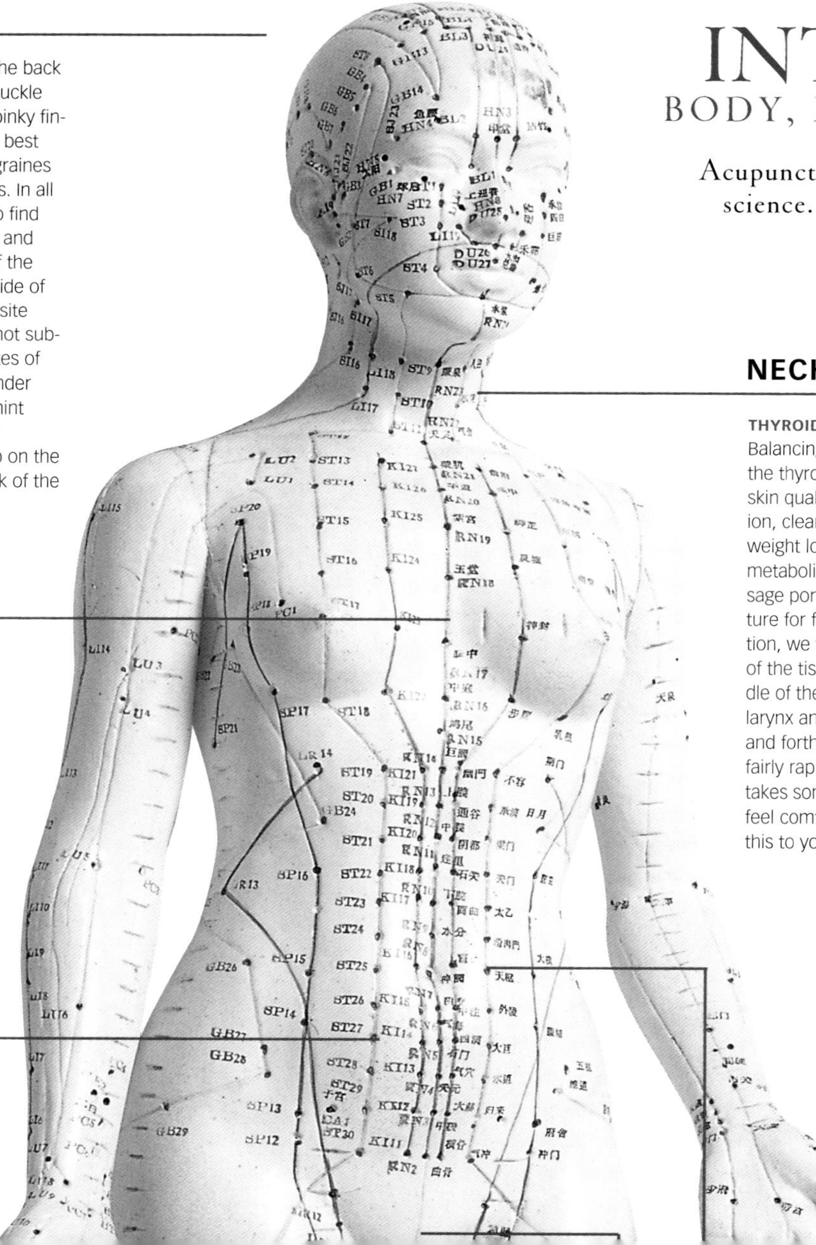

LUNG

LYMPH AND IMMUNE SYSTEM

Stimulating the left thoracic duct of the lymph system is an incredibly useful treatment to reduce a puffy face and help clear an infection that may be starting in the head, a sore throat, postnasal drip, or head congestion. Put the heel of your hand on the front of the chest under the clavicle bone, near the shoulder bone. This is also a lung point on the lung meridian. Rub the heel of your hand vigorously in circular motions for one to two minutes. The left side of the body is the most important one, but you can do the right side too if you like. This is a great technique for fighting off the very initial stages of a cold. Herbal and food remedies for fighting off the chill and congestion of a cold include miso soup with lots of fresh scallions and sliced or grated fresh ginger.

NECK

THYROID

Balancing the lobes of the thyroid can improve skin quality and complexion, clear acne, help weight loss, and improve metabolism. In the massage portion of acupuncture for facial rejuvenation, we firmly take hold of the tissue in the middle of the neck by the larynx and move it back and forth in a rhythmic, fairly rapid manner. It takes some practice to feel comfortable doing this to yourself. While stimulating the thyroid you should hum. Take a deep breath and hum while exhaling for several breaths. Doing this regularly stimulates and balances the two lobes of the thyroid. Herbs used in Chinese medicine to stimulate the thyroid include many of the seaweeds. You can find kombu in the health food store and use it in soups. You can also use dried beans or sprinkle other seaweeds like dulse or kelp on food.

STOMACH

NAUSEA

For stomach discomfort or nausea, there are two very effective areas of the body to stimulate with acupressure. One is on the lower leg, on the outside of the shinbone, where the bone begins to flare out near the knee. This may be a very tender point. Rub it gently but firmly to help combat nausea and fatigue. Another effective point that is a bit easier to reach is the inside of the forearm, in between the two tendons, about the distance of the width of three fingers up from the wrist. Again, rub this point gently but firmly to help fight nausea from motion sickness or morning sickness. A weak tea made from grated fresh ginger is also excellent for nausea. Or blend organic essential oils of ginger, lavender, and peppermint and breathe in the scent. Put a drop behind each ear.

BACK

LUMBAR PAIN

Find the point on the hand that's closer to the bone than the one recommended for frontal/sinus headaches. It's between the first finger and thumb, close to where the bones join together. This is usually very tender. Again, if your back hurts more on the left, concentrate primarily on stimulating the point on the right hand. Doing this can relieve a lot of lumbar discomfort. An effective herb used in Chinese medicinal teas is eucommia bark.

UTERUS

MENSTRUAL CRAMPS

To ease painful periods, you will find many tender points all along the inside of your shinbone, from the ankle to the knee. A point in the foot, in between the big toe and the second toe, may also be quite tender. All of these are great to massage. Cleaning up your diet is also key to reducing cramps: do not drink alcohol during your period, keep carbohydrates and processed foods to a minimum, and drink lots of water. Organic essential oils that can help are clary sage, lavender, fennel, marjoram, basil, and chamomile. Make a blend of a couple of drops of each in olive oil and rub on the lower back, the abdomen, and around the ankles.

Clean as You Go

In the professional kitchen, nothing is more important than *mise-en-place*. This classic French term (which literally means "put in place") refers to getting all the ingredients ready for use in a recipe. This means you won't get caught chopping the onion while you are burning the garlic that is already in the pan. If you can convert to this tried-and-true method, you will be amazed at how much easier it is to cook. The other golden rule to success in the preparation of food is the favorite motto of many chefs, "Clean as you go." This is vital. Psychologically it is much easier to cook because you don't always have in the back of your mind that everything must be cleaned up. Who wants to clean up everything after the meal has been eaten?

Start Fresh

The most important part of cooking is the ingredients that go into the final product. Always start with fresh, organic food. Food that is ripened fully before it is picked is that much better to eat. As Americans we need to learn to be pickier with our food and demand better quality. We are taught that "perfect" is shiny and round, but have you ever tasted a tomato, hot from sitting in the garden in the summer sun, sliced open and sprinkled with salt? Surely that bears no comparison to an agribusiness tomato that is crunchy and white inside with no flavor. There is something wrong if we are producing fruits and vegetables based on the mechanism that picks them, and not on their innate quality.

Buy Good Knives

At all costs no one should be without high-quality, sharp knives. I recommend starting with a paring knife and small eight-inch chef's knife. Almost anything can be done with these two essentials, but they must be kept sharp at all times. You have a better chance of cutting yourself with lesser-quality or dull knives than you do with professional-quality knives.

You Are What You Eat

It is so important to learn to cook basic, simple foods and to become less reliant on prepared foods and fast foods. What you eat directly affects your body and can affect it years down the road in the form of cancer and disease. Healthy, fresh food energizes you. Our bodies are such critical creatures yet we don't pay attention to the signals they give us. This doesn't mean you shouldn't enjoy food or subsist solely on rice crackers, but it means making the right choices and learning to be self-sufficient.

Read Recipes

Always read the entire thing through once. Then follow the instructions and ingredients carefully, making modifications only in future endeavors. Many people think that cooking always takes too much time, but by choosing simple recipes it doesn't have to. And it will be that much more satisfying that you cooked a meal yourself. Be confident that what you are cooking will be satisfying and delicious. Don't give up too quickly.

Cook, Eat, Enjoy

Cooking and eating should be enjoyable experiences. It should be as satisfying to cook for oneself as it is to cook for others and should never be a chore. The process of eating should be thought of as an experience no matter how simple or ornate the meal is. But it most certainly should not be forgotten or simply the background to whatever else is going on. After all, this is the stuff that keeps us going. As Elizabeth David said, a perfect meal can consist simply of "an omelet and a glass of wine."

Play with Your food

Experimenting while cooking is the real fun of cooking and where creativity comes into play. Yes, it is true that most cooks don't use recipes. We have practiced methods and techniques and experimented with flavors so many times that it becomes second nature. This comes to anyone in time. Listen to your taste buds. Have fun playing in the kitchen; cooking can be an art as much as it is a science. Don't be put off by the occasional disaster in the kitchen.

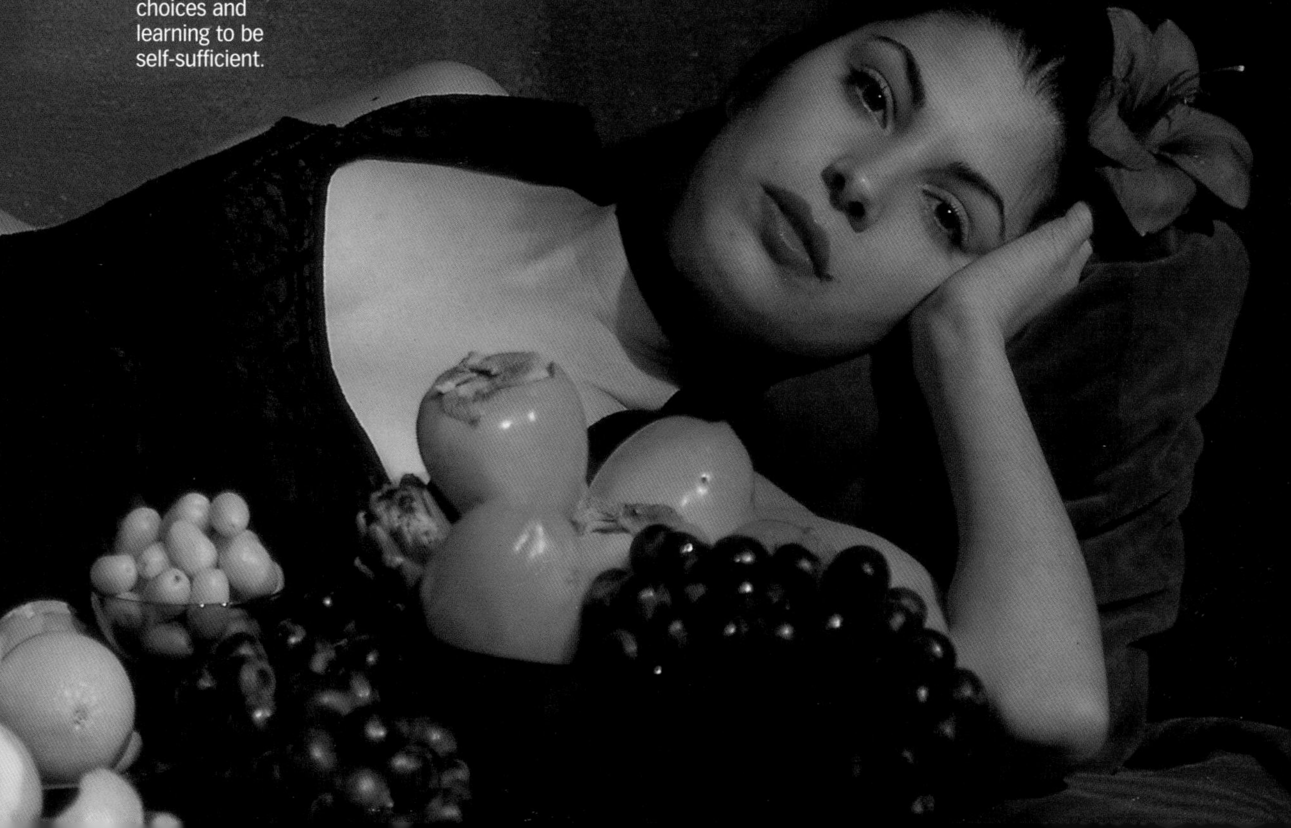

THERE IS A MAGIC
THAT OCCURS
WHEN WE TAKE THE TIME
TO BATHE IN
THE COMFORT
OF TAKING OUR MEALS
TOGETHER.

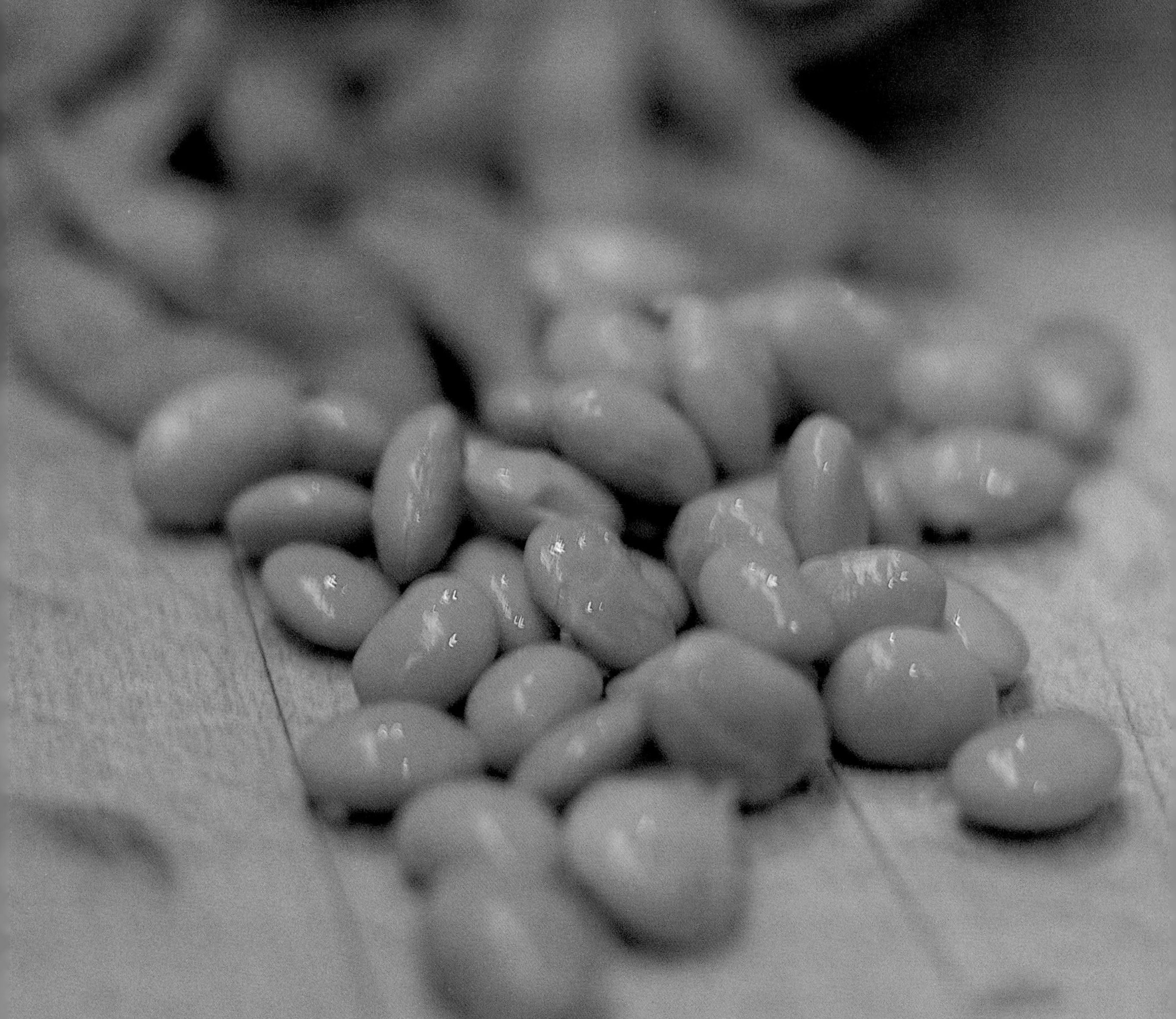

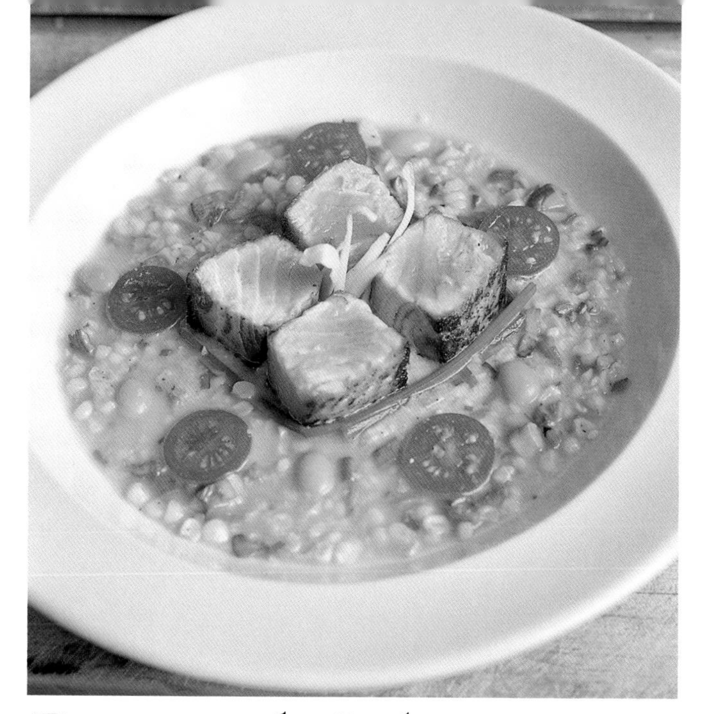

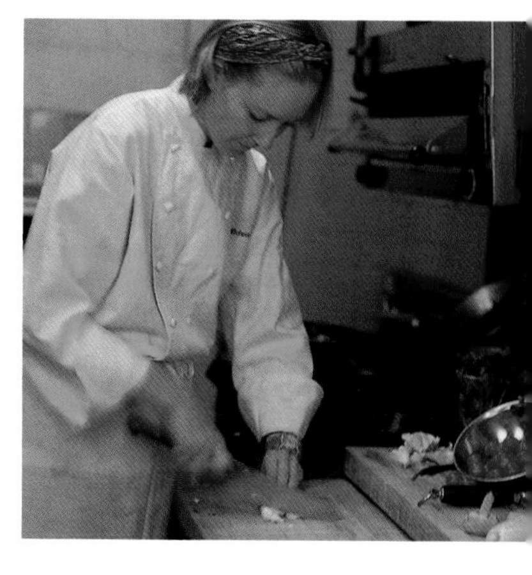

Roasted Salmon
with Fresh Soybean Puree

This is a wonderful combination of flavors and it's so good for you! Salmon is high in Omega-3 fatty acids, which are good for the heart, among other things. The soybeans are wonderful because they put phytoestrogens into your body. These compounds are said to decrease the effects of menopause (such as hot flashes) and prevent osteoporosis.

FOR THE PUREE:

2 cups fresh soybeans, blanched and shelled

1 tablespoon roughly chopped shallots

2 tablespoons rice wine

2 tablespoons soy oil

2 tablespoons roughly chopped cilantro or parsley

Salt and pepper to taste

FOR THE SALMON:

Soy oil as needed

1 tablespoon unsalted butter

1 tablespoon finely chopped shallots

1 cup diced oyster mushrooms

2 cups fresh corn cut off the cob

1 cup fresh soybeans, blanched and shelled

2 cups vegetable stock

10 cherry tomatoes, halved

Salt and pepper to taste

4 salmon fillets, 5 ounces each

4 teaspoons finely chopped cilantro or parsley

To make the puree, combine the soybeans, shallots, rice wine, oil, and cilantro in a blender and puree until smooth and thick. Season to taste with salt and pepper. It may be necessary to add a small amount of warm water to achieve the right consistency. Set aside. (This may be made ahead of time. It is delicious chilled as a dip, too.)

To make the salmon, heat a sauté pan and coat the bottom with a thin layer of oil. Add the butter, shallots, and mushrooms and sauté until softened, about 2 minutes. Add the corn and soybeans and cook for 1 minute. Add the stock, bring to a simmer, and add the tomatoes. Season to taste with salt and pepper. (This should be made just before the salmon is cooked.)

Heat another sauté pan and coat the bottom with a thin layer of oil. Season both sides of the salmon fillets with salt and pepper. Add salmon to the smoking hot pan. Cook for about 2 minutes on each side or longer if desired.

To serve, place soybean puree in the centers of 4 individual serving bowls. Slice each fillet into 4 pieces and arrange them in the puree with the center of the fish facing up. Surround the salmon with the vegetable broth garnish. Sprinkle salmon with salt.

SERVINGS: 4

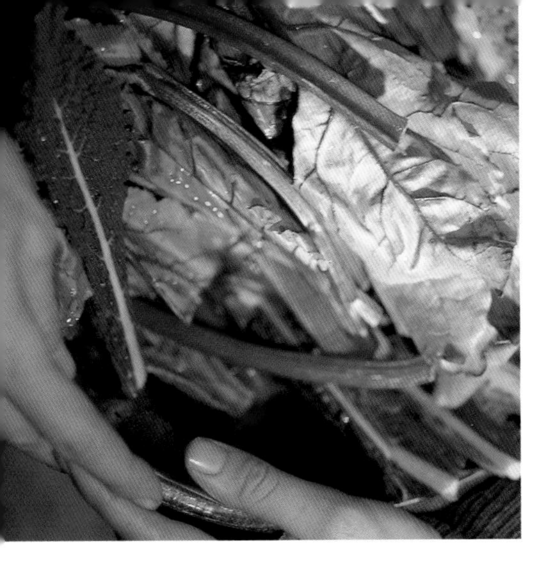

Hearty Vegetable Soup for Weight Control

Soups are one of the most versatile, comforting, satisfying, and basic foods. In this one we have included a base broth utilizing Chinese herbs that promote weight loss and lowering of cholesterol. We call for scallions and kale but any greens will do—beet greens would be a great substitute. As a guide, look for seasonal produce and add it in the later stages of cooking, allowing just enough time for the vegetable to cook. This soup is particularly good for women who normally feel abdominal distention after eating and tend to be a bit tired or feel sluggish.

What it tastes like: Most people are put off by the idea of eating the unknown. This soup has wonderful flavor and texture. In fact, the Chinese herbs do not impart any strong flavors. It is an incredibly nutritive and delicious soup. It is recommended that you eat 2 to 4 cups a day for at least one week for maximum benefit.

- 2 ounces astragalus root
- 2 ounces poria fungus
- 1/2 ounce rehydrated black fungus, broken into pieces
- 12 red dates, rehydrated and pitted
- 1/4 cup finely chopped fresh ginger
- 1 cup barley
- 3 quarts vegetable or chicken stock
- 1 1/2 cups diced celery
- 3 beets, cut into strips
- 1 1/2 cups sliced shiitake mushrooms
- 3 cloves garlic, finely chopped
- 8 cups kale, very roughly chopped
- 1 bunch scallions, sliced
- 1/2 cup finely chopped parsley
- Salt to taste

Place the astragalus in a muslin bag or tie with a string. Simmer the astragalus, poria, black fungus, red dates, ginger, and barley in the stock for 1 hour. Add the celery, beets, shiitake mushrooms, garlic, and kale and cook for another 20 minutes. Remove the astragalus. Add scallions and parsley. Season to taste with salt. Add more water if necessary for consistency. Cook for 2 minutes more.

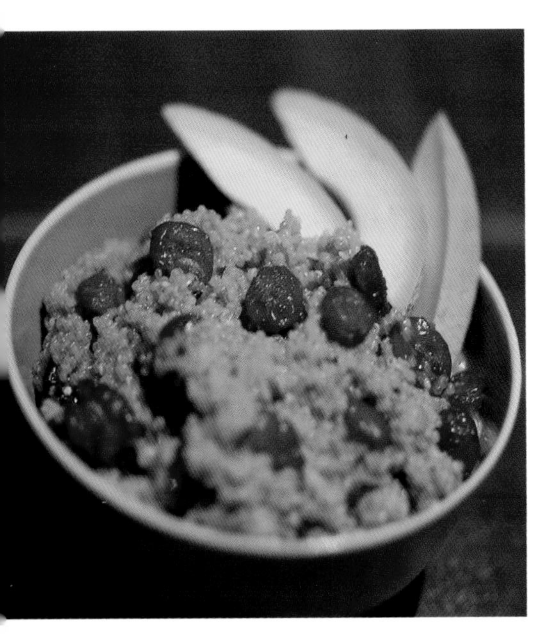

Fruited Mint and Basil Quinoa Salad for Health

- 1/2 cup roughly chopped mint
- 1 1/2 cups roughly chopped basil
- 1/2 cup shelled pistachios
- 1/2 cup grated Parmigiano Reggiano cheese
- 2 tablespoons balsamic vinegar
- 1/2 cup olive oil
- 3/4 cup dried organic, unsulphured apricots
- 3/4 cup dried cranberries
- 4 cups quinoa, cooked per package directions and drained of any excess liquid
- Salt and pepper to taste

Combine the mint, basil, pistachios, cheese, vinegar, and olive oil in a blender and puree until a grainy paste is achieved, adding warm water if necessary. Season to taste with salt and pepper. Add the apricots and cranberries to this mixture and let sit for at least half an hour. Toss with the quinoa. Season to taste. YIELD: 1 quart

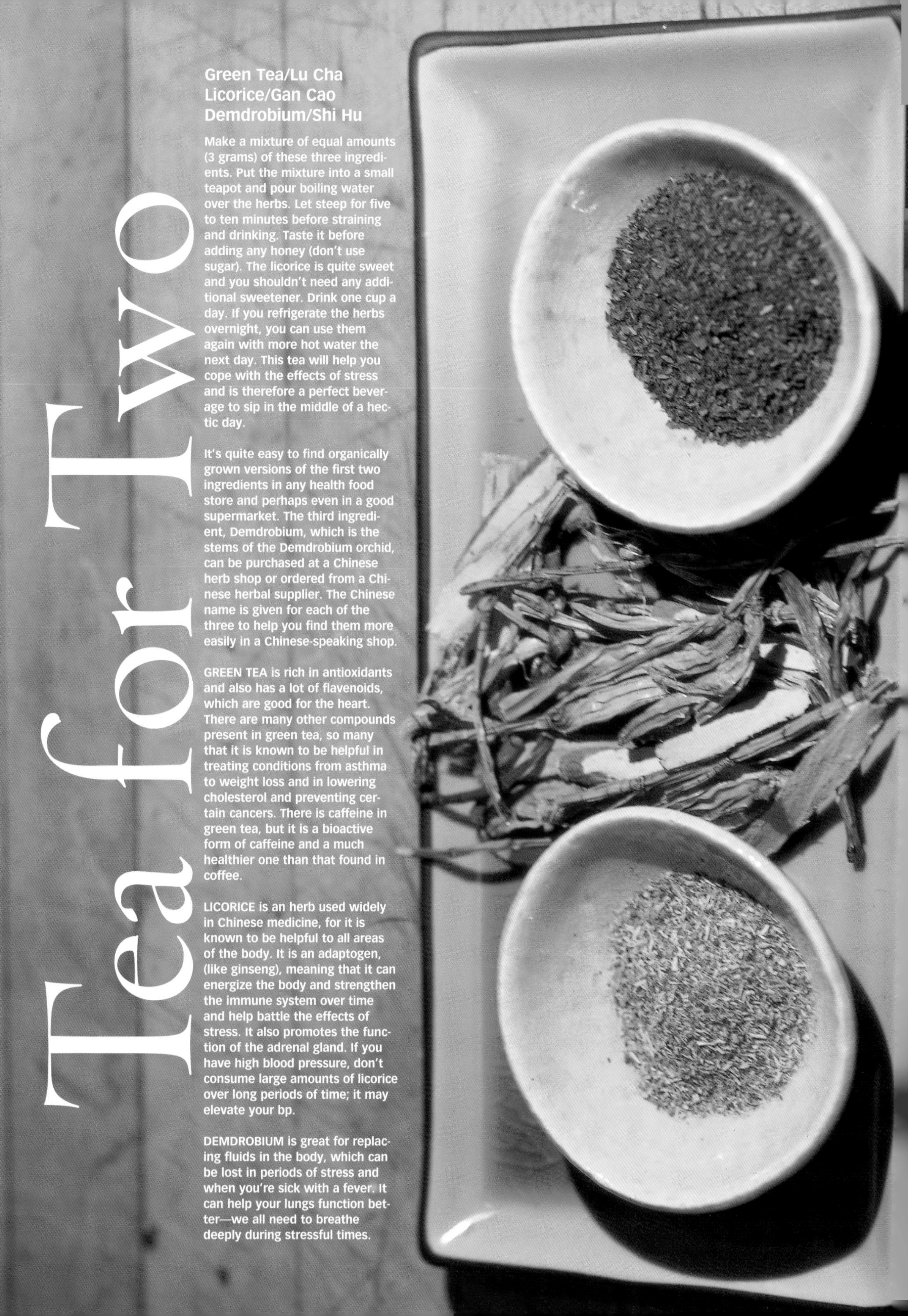

Tea for Two

Green Tea/Lu Cha
Licorice/Gan Cao
Demdrobium/Shi Hu

Make a mixture of equal amounts (3 grams) of these three ingredients. Put the mixture into a small teapot and pour boiling water over the herbs. Let steep for five to ten minutes before straining and drinking. Taste it before adding any honey (don't use sugar). The licorice is quite sweet and you shouldn't need any additional sweetener. Drink one cup a day. If you refrigerate the herbs overnight, you can use them again with more hot water the next day. This tea will help you cope with the effects of stress and is therefore a perfect beverage to sip in the middle of a hectic day.

It's quite easy to find organically grown versions of the first two ingredients in any health food store and perhaps even in a good supermarket. The third ingredient, Demdrobium, which is the stems of the Demdrobium orchid, can be purchased at a Chinese herb shop or ordered from a Chinese herbal supplier. The Chinese name is given for each of the three to help you find them more easily in a Chinese-speaking shop.

GREEN TEA is rich in antioxidants and also has a lot of flavenoids, which are good for the heart. There are many other compounds present in green tea, so many that it is known to be helpful in treating conditions from asthma to weight loss and in lowering cholesterol and preventing certain cancers. There is caffeine in green tea, but it is a bioactive form of caffeine and a much healthier one than that found in coffee.

LICORICE is an herb used widely in Chinese medicine, for it is known to be helpful to all areas of the body. It is an adaptogen, (like ginseng), meaning that it can energize the body and strengthen the immune system over time and help battle the effects of stress. It also promotes the function of the adrenal gland. If you have high blood pressure, don't consume large amounts of licorice over long periods of time; it may elevate your bp.

DEMDROBIUM is great for replacing fluids in the body, which can be lost in periods of stress and when you're sick with a fever. It can help your lungs function better—we all need to breathe deeply during stressful times.

VERNA MOSES

Fitness instructor Verna Moses, **an avid cyclist, has been teaching spinning in New York for more than six years.** Her spinning career was purely accidental; as a graduate of law school, she never envisioned that she would pursue a career that did not require her to wear panty hose. Her technical and uniquely motivational style of instruction–infused with a dash of humor–have brought her a cult following, and she now teaches more than twenty classes a week to an audience of thousands. She says, "it has been a wonderful, exciting, and totally unexpected ride. I am honored to have been able to touch so many lives." Verna and her class have been recognized in such national publications as *Self* and *Vogue*. She is currently preparing to take the New York Bar Exam and to bring her unique style of teaching to Europe. She is also working on Body FX, a new and innovative line of clothing and accessories.

Q Your work centers on keeping people focused and driven to achieve their goals. Given what you have learned in your career as a fitness instructor, what words of wisdom would you pass on to other women?

Be happy honoring yourself. Schedule alone-time for you and nurture your core self. The best possible gift that you could ever give someone is you, healthy and happy. From there, everything else will fall into place. It will affect the way you look, act, and deal with personal relationships, and even the depth of your soul. And don't be afraid to take chances. Women so often live someone else's dream or are willing to work on the things that other people want to do. But with their own dreams they often think only of the reasons why they shouldn't do it, that maybe they're not good enough or

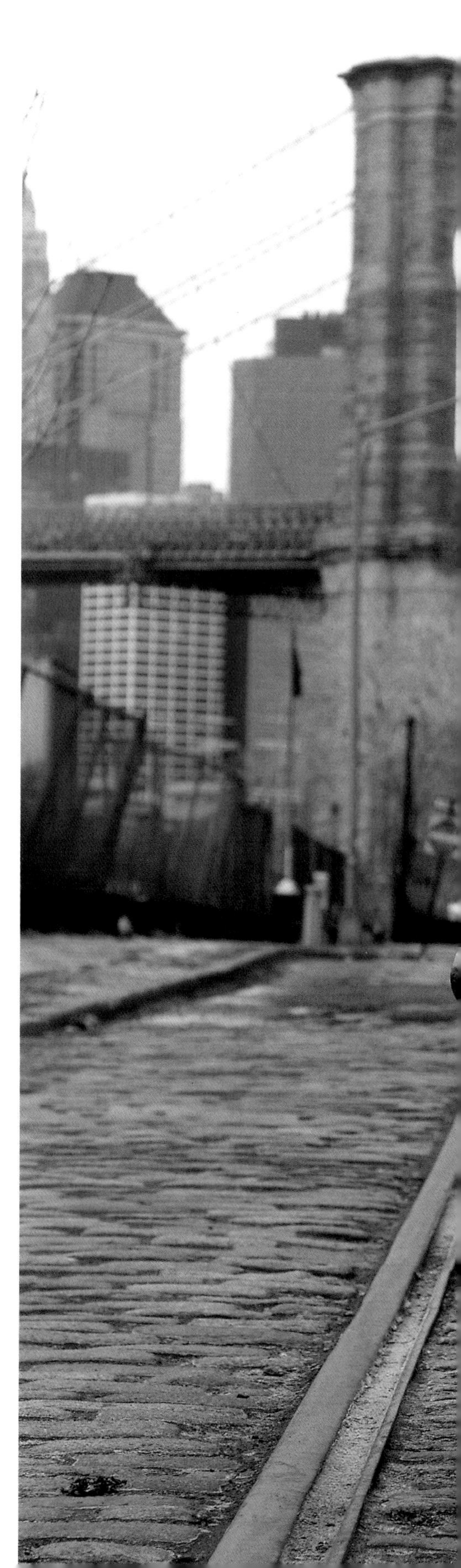

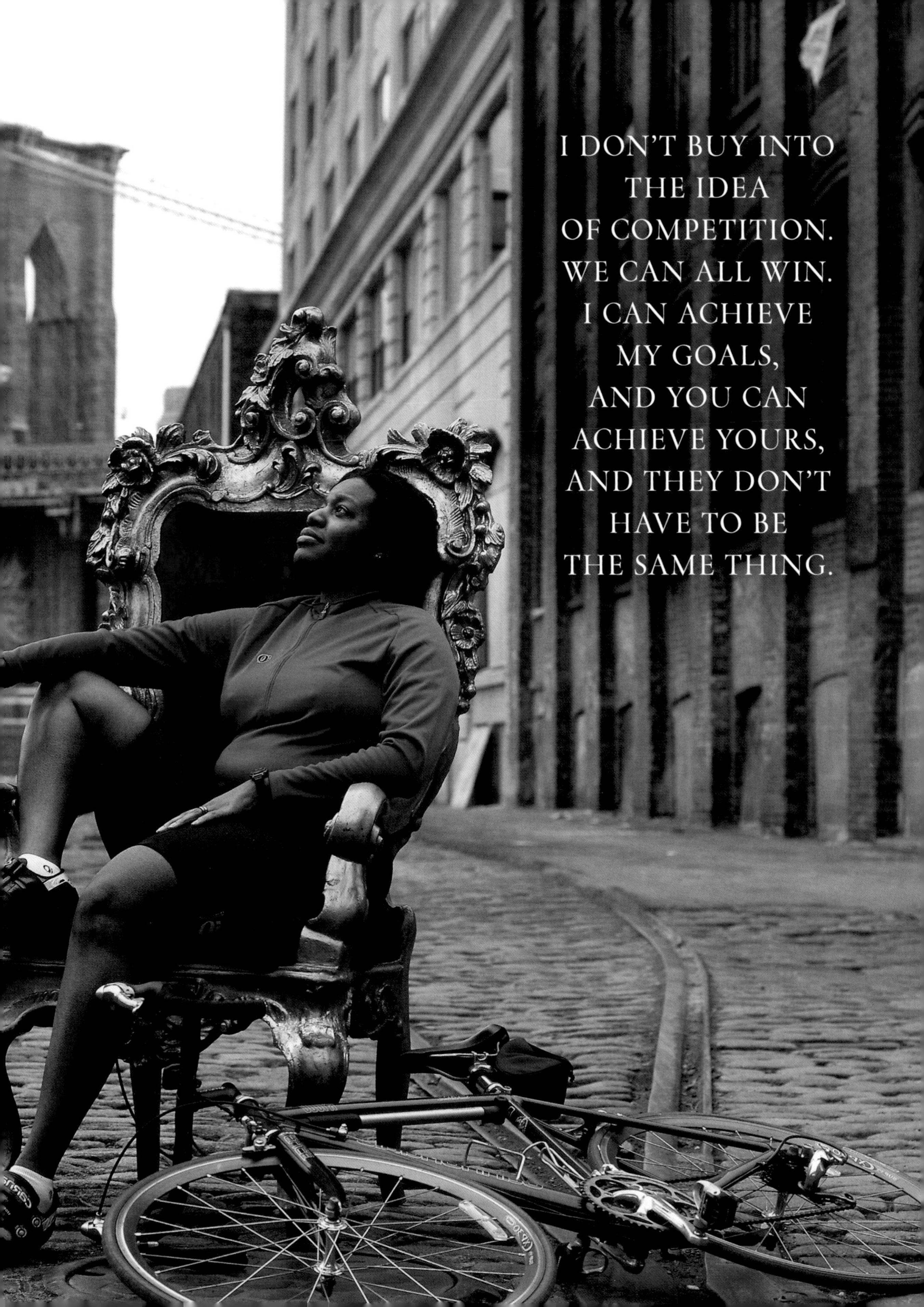
I DON'T BUY INTO
THE IDEA
OF COMPETITION.
WE CAN ALL WIN.
I CAN ACHIEVE
MY GOALS,
AND YOU CAN
ACHIEVE YOURS,
AND THEY DON'T
HAVE TO BE
THE SAME THING.

that it's too competitive out there. But who better to take a chance on than yourself? The worst that could happen is you fail. But in the end, you always learn something and you're stronger for having tried. And stop worrying about what other people think.

Q I understand you had a rather bumpy ride on the road to becoming a top fitness instructor. You started your professional life as a lawyer—was law a great passion of yours?

I was the first in my family to go to college. I was raised by my mother, who gave me a lot of love and encouragement, but I had no academic role models as a child. I just got it in my mind that I was going to do something none of the people around me had done. So after high school I attended Spellman, a black women's college. And from there I went to law school.

Then, during the summer after my final year in law school, I was given the opportunity to be an intern at a large firm in Maryland. This was a dream. Out of thirteen summer associates, only three of us were accepted. At the end of every summer they kept one person on as an employee, and that year they chose me. I was the first black woman to receive an offer from this firm–that was mind-blowing for me. I never thought that I would be the first anything. But working there made me miserable. I was forced into the employment discrimination department, and it became clear to me that I was being used as a token. I would wake up each day and before my feet hit the floor I was holding my face, full of tears. After three months, I'd had it. I went home for the holidays and never went back. I decided that there was no reason for me to be so unhappy.

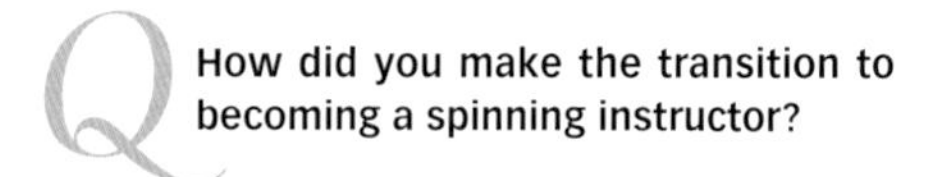

Q How did you make the transition to becoming a spinning instructor?

Fast-forward two and a half years, during which time I cared for my aunt and uncle, who had fallen ill. I was still unhappy, but I couldn't leave them. I knew that I had to get out of the miserable rut I was in, so I decided to dance. I started looking for a hip-hop class and finally found one at a gym in Manhattan. To get to the gym, I started commuting the ten miles by bicycle. Then I heard they were looking for spinning instructors. My main motivation was a free gym membership. I knew I could do it, but my big concern was how I would make it interesting for me. The spinning that was being taught at that time was very meditative and not my style at all. The people at the gym were very supportive of me and I knew it would be great if I just found a way to put myself into the class. It was the first thing I had been passionate about for so many years. I finally felt like I had found my niche.

I started with one class on Friday nights at a funky downtown gym. I had attended only two classes myself, so at first it was horrible. I was uncomfortable and unsure of myself. But soon I was in a groove and began to build quite a following. I've been doing it for six years now, teaching more than twenty classes a week. And I've never been happier.

Q Why do you think that women are attracted to your classes?

Everyone is special in my class. They are encouraged to just begin where they are and progress from there. I remember each person's name or I give them a name. Women really respond to that personal attention. Women also respond well to positive reinforcement, especially where our bodies and athleticism are concerned. And it just comes naturally to me to be really excited about someone accomplishing their goal, no matter what it is. I also make sure to break things down–like the technical cycling terms or the way that we're supposed to be pedaling–to their basic elements so they are easier to understand and not too overwhelming. Women are great at being open to instruction. They're not too wrapped up in their egos to say that they don't understand what I am talking about. And it's really rewarding for me to be able to teach them something that will put them in touch with their bodies or allow them to understand a more efficient riding technique. I think it also works well because I feed off their energy. The response I get from women really keeps me going. One woman told me I was better than Prozac. They tell me I uplift them, but many times I feel it's them uplifting me.

Q What do you consider the style of your classes?

Motivational. What I say in class is the same thing I say to myself when I am working out. "Give it up to the feeling," or "It's okay if you are hurting right now, just release it." It's

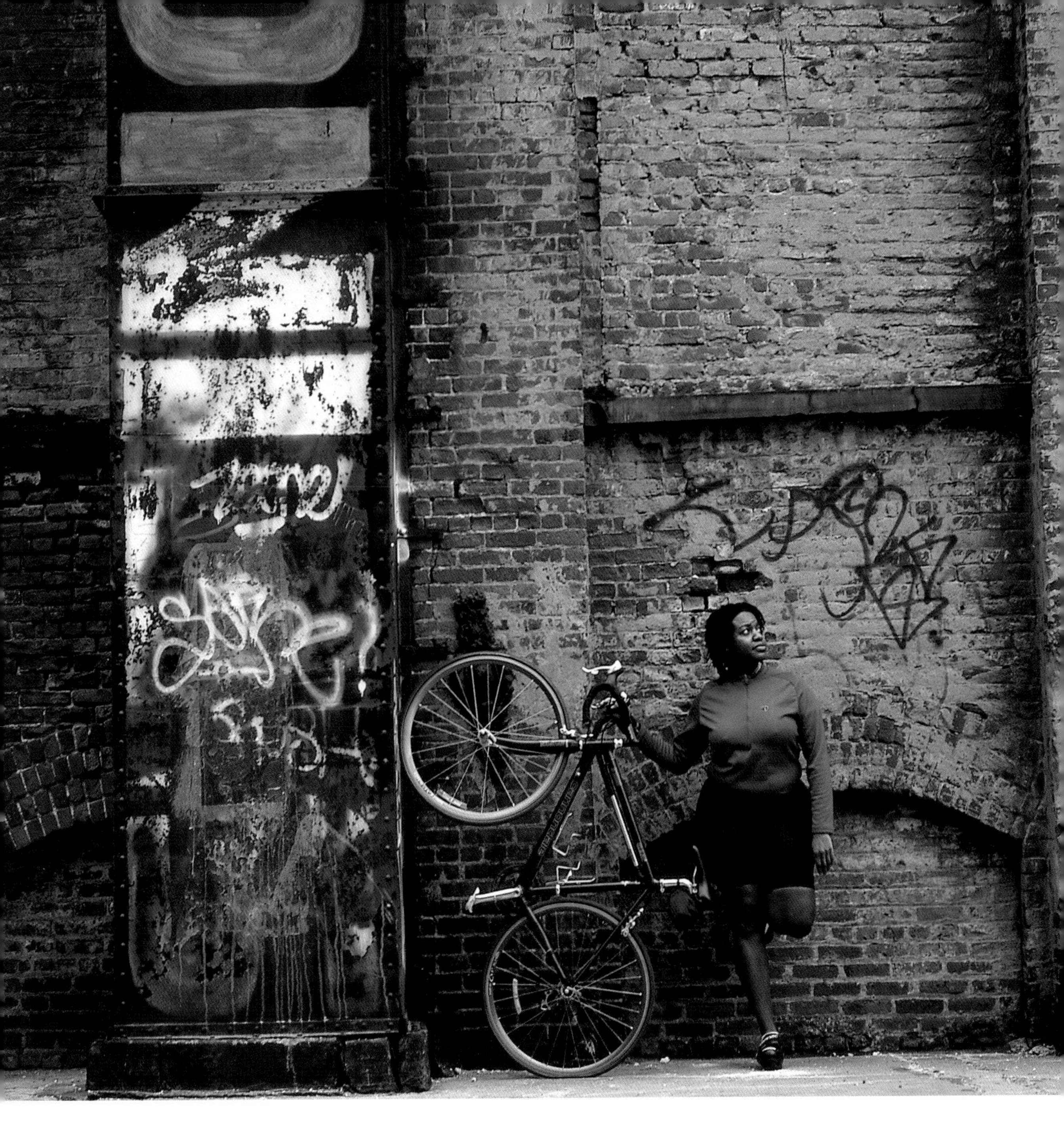

okay to make noise. It doesn't need to be pretty. The music is also a big part of the atmosphere. I choose songs with good cadence and snippets of motivational ideas in the lyrics like "Your eyes can't believe what your mind can't conceive." Humor is also important. Workouts don't have to be serious all the time. Too much seriousness and pressure on yourself takes all the pleasure out of it. There needs to be some levity because–wow–it can really hurt! So laugh! Let it out! Before you know it, you've achieved your goal and you feel great. I don't buy into the idea of competition. I believe the only one you have to compete with is yourself. We can all win. I can achieve my goals, you can achieve yours, and they don't have to be the same thing.

I always make sure to track people's progress because I am excited to see them reaching their goals. So many people go through life thinking that no one notices or cares, but that caring and interest comes naturally to me. I'm not making it up. I teach my classes from the heart.

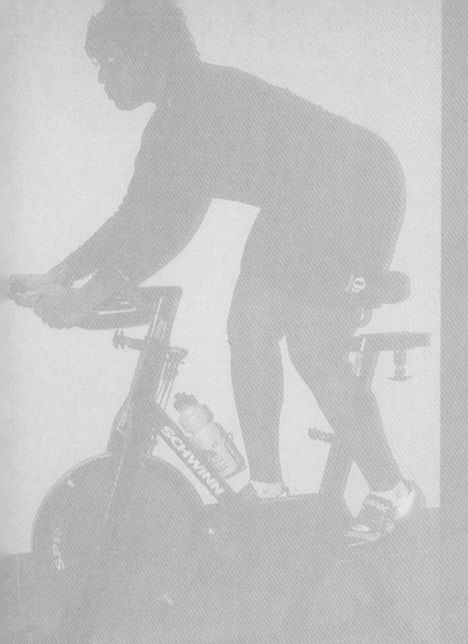

Cycle to Your Health!
A Few Healthy Reasons to Just Do It

In my opinion, cycling—on the road or off—is one of the greatest exercises for women. The women that I spin and road cycle with express the same feelings. Riding makes them feel excited, uplifted, strengthened, fulfilled, contented, and energized. Cycling evokes a sense of freedom and purpose, and because of the solo nature of the sport, it gives busy women a chance to reflect in a meditative way. Plus, the health benefits are tremendous. So if you don't cycle, you should. And if you do, then cycle more!

Cycling and Weight Control

The rate of calorie burning in cycling is almost unsurpassed. One hour of intense cycling can burn anywhere from 400 to 800 calories! (Needless to say, food deprivation is not only an unhealthy way to lose weight; it is also unnecessary for the cyclist who follows a healthy diet.)

Ride Back from Depression

Regular doses of exercise using the large muscle groups in regular rhythm appear to produce chemical and physiological changes in the body and brain that will affect the mood. Regular cycling, along with good nutrition, promotes homeostasis—the body's own natural propensity to balance its own chemistry.

Overcoming Substance Abuse

Fitness is not merely the key to recovery—it's often the missing link. There is no health problem in which the mind and body are more connected than substance abuse. Cycling brings back the feeling of control that has been lost in one's life. Exercise is also one of the greatest weapons for fighting cravings—food and cigarettes included.

A Healthier Heart

To stay out of the high-risk category, women should start exercising prior to menopause to minimize the rise in cholesterol as they age. Exercise such as cycling reduces cholesterol and increases the percentage of the beneficial HDL. It also helps combat high blood pressure, which can ultimately lead to heart disease and kidney failure.

Protection Against Cancer

Body fat converts androgens to estrogen. There is a lower cancer rate among people with lower levels of estrogen due to exercise. Studies confirm a protective effect for those who become active later in life.

Dodging Diabetes

Along with a proper diet, the benefits of regular exercise in managing and avoiding all types of diabetes have been well documented. Moderate exercise assists by taking some of the glucose out of the blood and using it for energy, which keeps blood glucose levels normal. If you do have diabetes, cycling offers the right kind of exercise for the disorder.

Some Verna-isms: Your eyes won't believe what your mind can't conceive. If you believe it, you can achieve it. Up and down, round and round . . . like pistons, baby. You can make it . . . I know you can, I know you will. You have determination in your eyes and confidence in your heart. Let nothing block your way, because this is your day. You've come too far to turn back now. (Push) harder, (go) faster, (spin) longer. Keep breathing, no grieving, soon you will be leaving.

CYCLING FOR THE BEGINNER

Choose a bicycle that is appropriate for the riding you intend to do. In addition to different sizes, bicycles also differ in type (road, touring, hybrid, and mountain). Visit a reputable bike shop to be measured and discuss your cycling goals. Don't be intimidated; bike salesmen should not employ high-pressure sales tactics.

Wear a helmet. Just as you would never go cycling without your clothes, don't leave your head naked either. A helmet protects the essence of who you are.

Bring a tool kit. Unfortunately, there's no AAA for cyclists. Pack a spare tube or patch kit, tire levers, a pump, Allen wrenches, a Phillips-head screwdriver, and an adjustable wrench. Most of these tools can be purchased in a compact all-in-one kit at a bike shop.

Make sure the ball of your foot is on the pedal, not your arch or heel. Also, keep the foot heading relatively straight ahead while pedaling.

Relax the shoulders and keep your elbows and wrists in the proper position. The body acts much the same as a shock absorber in a car. Proper positioning will help you avoid joint and upper back problems in the future.

SPINNING FOR THE BEGINNER

Inform the instructor that you are new and mention any physical conditions that you have. The instructor should then set you up on a bike in the proper position.

Familiarize yourself with the braking system. Because the spin bike is a fixed-gear bike it will require a certain amount of expertise to stop the bike with your feet. Learn how to use the brake! It could prevent serious injury.

Focus on your form: relax your shoulders, bend your elbows slightly, and keep your knees in alignment with your feet. This includes keeping your hands on the handlebars at all times during a ride.

Bring water, a towel, and stiff-soled shoes. You do not need a shoe that absorbs impact, like you do in aerobics. You need a shoe that provides a proper barrier between your foot and the pedal.

No matter how small or large the derriere may be, most will find the seat uncomfortable. Accept it, embrace it, and know that this feeling will pass. In the meantime, you can wear a pair of cycling shorts made specifically for women. There are also soft gel seat covers.

Work within your fitness level. Initially your motto should be, "Live to spin another day!" Remember that the pyramids were not built in a day. You will not be able to master cycling in a day or even a month. Focus on each of your milestones and your success will be imminent.

DR. CAROLYN DEAN

IT IS MY MISSION TO WORK TOWARD A LARGER VISION OF WHAT MEDICINE CAN BE IN PEOPLE'S LIVES.

Alternative physician Dr. Carolyn Dean, with her unique combination of a medical degree and naturopathic degree, began practicing complementary integrative medicine in 1979. Her current projects include writing about digital disease and media ecology; inventing new technology for the herb industry; writing a book on food therapy with Jeffrey Yuen, a Taoist priest and Chinese medicine scholar; and acting as a spokesperson and consultant for *Natural Health* magazine and Weider Publications. A true visionary, she has always understood that a doctor is really a teacher and in 1994 she self-published one of the first encyclopedias on the practical use of herbs, homeopathy, and nutrition. *Complementary Natural Prescriptions for Common Ailments* is now in its second revision with Keats Publishing. Carolyn's educational role spills into other media and she is a contributor to such television programs as *The View*, bringing joy and humor into health education.

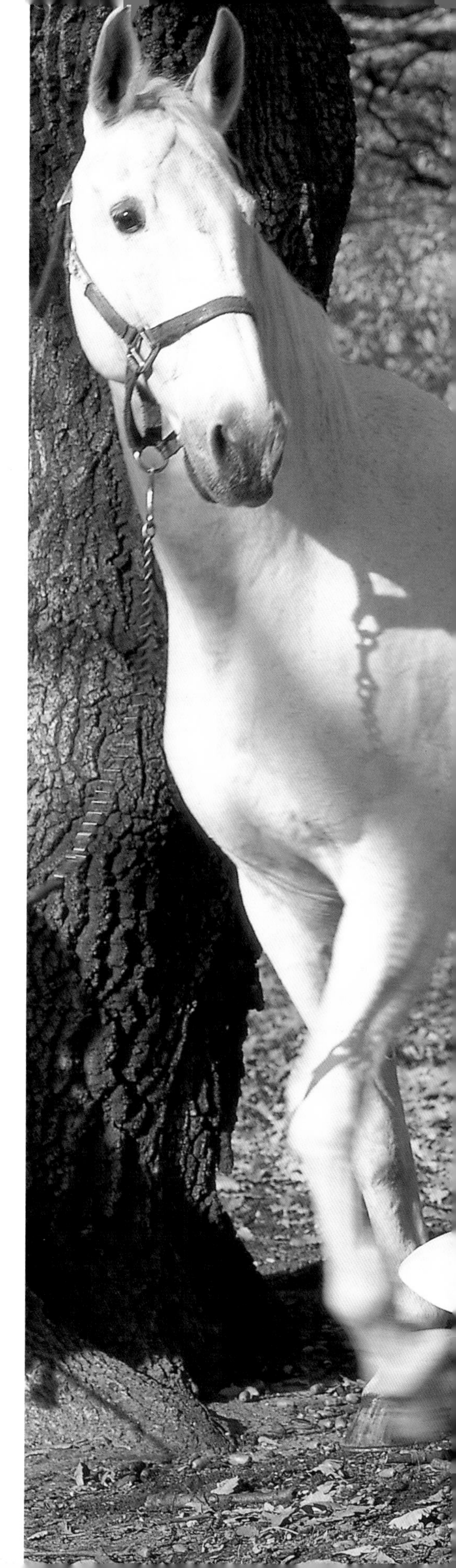

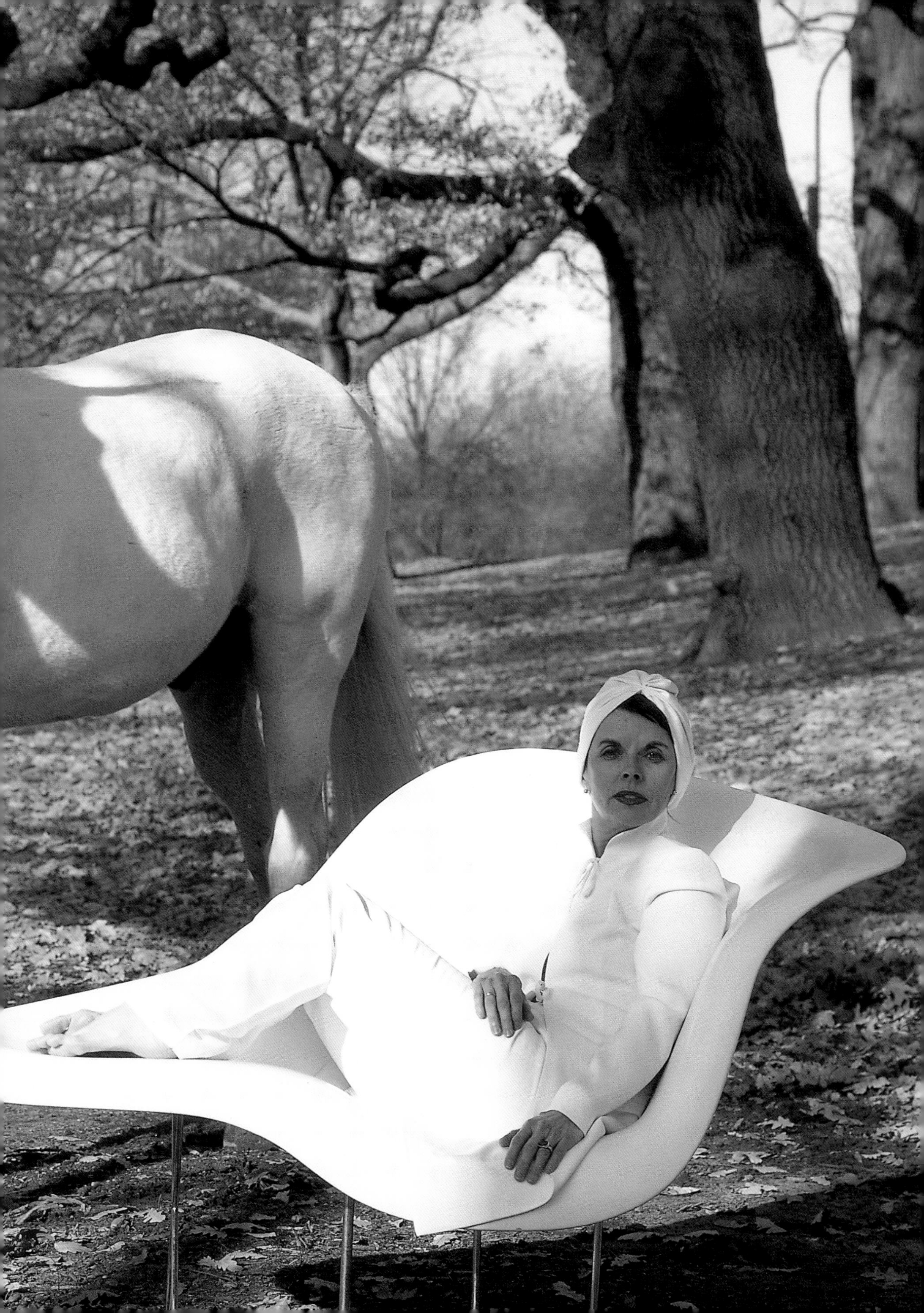

Q Medical school in the early seventies must have been a real boys' club. Less than 25 percent of the people attending at that time were women. What was it like to be among them?

I just made it really plain that I was there to be a great doctor and I wasn't going to be overlooked or dismissed. My school was definitely white-male oriented, and its treatment of women inspired me to make my presence felt on several occasions. I remember on the second day of class a clinician came in to give a slide presentation. His second or third slide was a pornographic picture of a nude female. He said he did it to keep the mens' attention. The women in the class all hissed and rumbled but nobody said anything. So I took action. *Playgirl* had just come out, so I bought a copy, cut out a male nude pin-up, and had a slide made that I snuck into the clinician's slide tray two days later. When it was projected onto the screen, everyone was shocked. That put an end to that.

Another time, we had a pediatrician come in and talk about breast-feeding versus bottle-feeding. He was saying that bottle-feeding was just fine, no better or worse than breast-feeding. By coincidence, I had just read some research stating that breast-feeding had been proven to be better than bottle-feeding. So I said to him, "Excuse me, sir, there is this study that shows that, in fact, breast-feeding is superior to bottle-feeding." Immediately he responded to me with, "Oh, Bubbles, what do you know?" Isn't that amazing?

Q I bet that those experiences drove you even harder into your passion for enlightening the medical world. With so much pressure, how you did you manage to go the extra mile and incorporate alternative medicine into your curriculum?

It is my mission to work toward a larger vision of what medicine can be in people's lives. In one of my second-year electives, I arranged to study acupuncture with one of the only Chinese doctors who did acupuncture in Halifax. Mind you, I was the only one who did it. Then when I got my internship, I actually started practicing and showing acupuncture to new students when we were doing clinical rounds, which was unheard of. I was also learning homeopathy, herbal medicine, and Chinese medicine. My peers thought I was crazy, but I just brushed it off.

Q What type of support system did you have during all of this? I understand that alternative medicine is in your blood.

I was born in Newfoundland, but I grew up in Dartmouth, Nova Scotia. My mother had become a nurse in Scotland before she moved to North America with my father. The training there involved a lot of natural medicine and common sense. In fact, she had a reputation in our local community for helping anyone who came to her. My dad's mother was also a nurse and a homeopath and a healer. Her work in the field reached back to the beginning of the century.

My father was slated to be a doctor. He was entered in Harvard Medical School when his father got sick. His family had to move up north, and he became responsible for taking care of them. He could no longer attend school and Harvard became out of the question.

I applied to medical school because there were no alternative medicine schools anywhere in Canada. And even medical school seemed almost

Media Moderation

Be aware of the pervasiveness of the media and the electronic environment. Antidote TV and the Internet with a good book and some music. Try to take regular "media fasts."

Use Discernment

Be discerning about the information you gather and try not to be swayed by extreme views and belief systems. Bottom line for me is: "Who funded the research or article and who benefits from the results?" Follow the money! Consult the original source directly.

Watch Your Diet

Be sure your diet includes organic vegetables and fruits; antibiotic-free, hormone-free meats; soaked, sprouted, fermented grains; organic yogurt; butter, flax oil, olive oil, and coconut oil; minimal sugar and desserts; no artificial sweeteners; natural (nonsynthetic) supplements. Join or create an organic co-op and order wholesale organic goods.

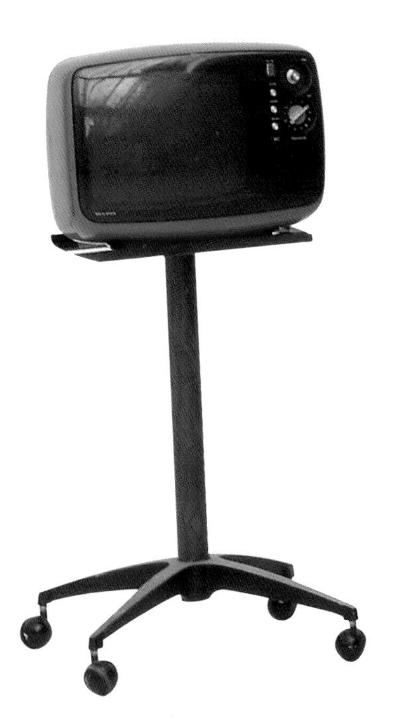

SUBSTITUTE TV AND THE INTERNET WITH A GOOD BOOK AND GOOD MUSIC AND TRY TO TAKE REGULAR "MEDIA FASTS."

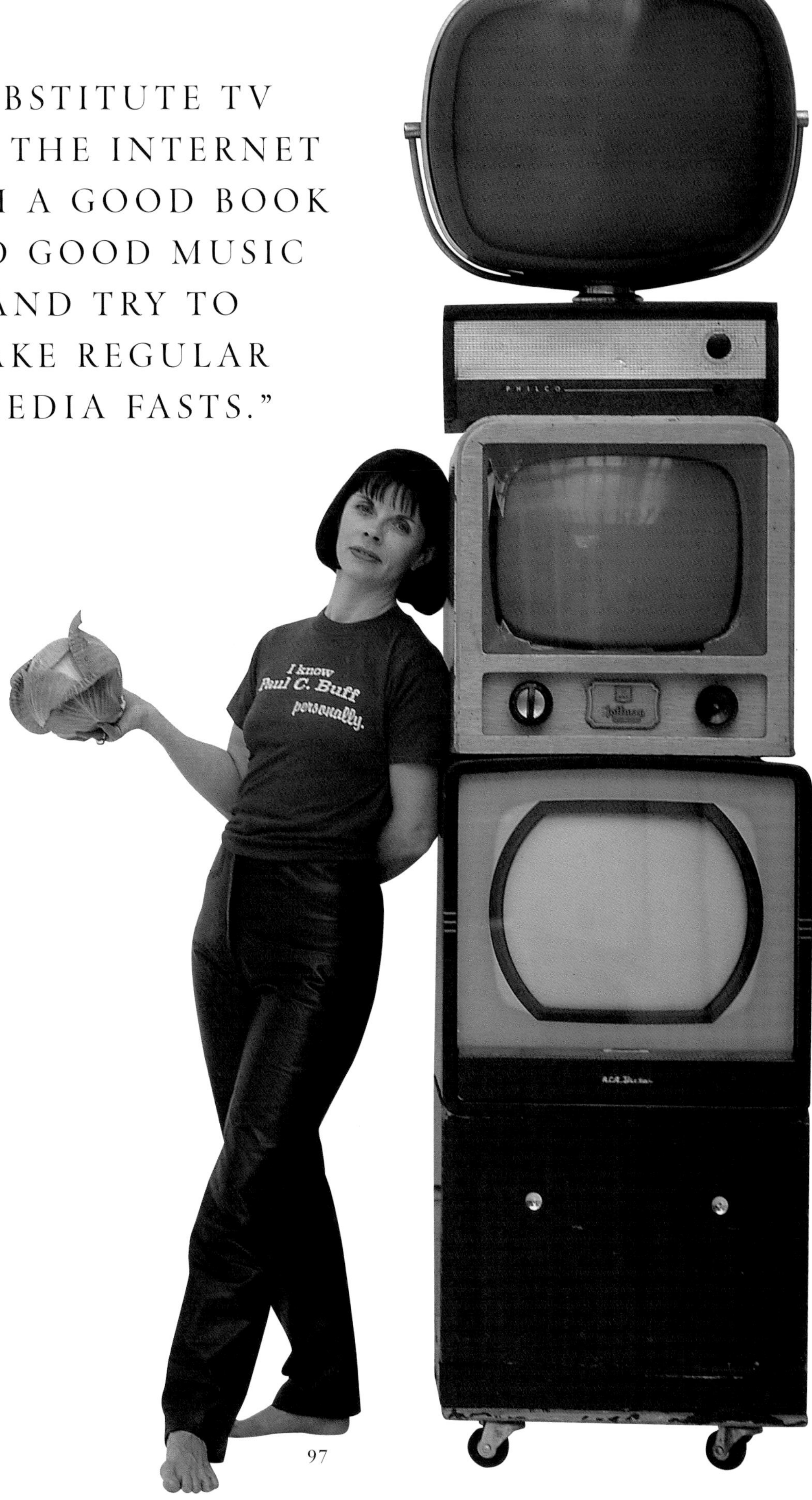

Creative Control

Practice creative control over your life: affirm what you want, then create opportunities to achieve your goals. I believe we attract what we vibrate or emanate. If we project good thoughts and perform the right actions, we will attract the same to us.

Stick to Your Principles

Don't compromise your principles. Try to speak your mind when you first perceive a problem with someone. But apologize just as quickly if you are in the wrong.

out of reach because of my gender. In fact, at my admissions interview I remember asking Dr. Nicholson, the dean of students, "What are the chances of me getting in? I'm tiny, almost deaf, and a woman." To the tiny he responded, "Carolyn, you may look small, but you don't sound small." About the deafness he said, "Most students don't listen anyway." And as for my being a woman he said, "We're getting applications from very qualified women like yourself and it's about time we started accepting more of them."

My second interview was with third-year medical students. They rejected my application because I was too optimistic about what could be done in medicine. Dr. Nicholson and I had a great laugh over that one and he said one day I would do great things for medicine.

When I told my folks that I'd been accepted to medical school, my father got this odd look on his face and kind of turned pale and told me his story. It brings a tear to my eye even today to think that I am living his dream as well as mine.

Q Once you graduated from medical school, was it difficult to gain respect as an alternative doctor? Judging from the reaction you received from other students, I can only imagine what the general public thought.

Actually, the public was hungry for an alternative doctor. With all of the training I made sure I got while in school, I was actually able to start using natural medicine the first day I opened my doors, and I had one of the fastest-growing practices in Toronto. Word of mouth that I was doing alternative medicine spread like wildfire. I was happily swamped. Then, because what I was doing was unique for a medical doctor, people started asking me to do lectures. That led to other media, radio, and TV.

On a national talk show I did in 1989, I was talking about sugar and showing the audience how much is contained in certain common foods (eight teaspoons in a soda, twenty-five teaspoons in a milkshake—that sort of thing). Not long after, a sugar-lobby group complained about me to the College of Physicians and Surgeons (CPSO). They were upset that I was saying bad things about sugar. I found out later that the CPSO was watching and systematically investigating all the alternative medicine doctors and trying to suppress our work. Luckily I avoided most of the high drama because I went off on a sabbatical that I had planned for several years to avoid burnout. I came to New York to work on a project and ended up staying.

At the same time, the investigation of alternative medicine doctors by the CPSO escalated. Ironically, their crusade backfired and turned into a reverse investigation. The College of Physicians and Surgeons is now being investigated by the government for inappropriate criminal activity against alternative medicine doctors. You see, a lot of people in the medical profession are on the boards of various drug companies. Alternative practitioners do nothing but lower drug sales, and the sugar thing was just an excuse to investigate me. It does seem odd to be part of this huge scandal. But when you're on the cutting edge, it can get a little bloody.

Q There have been a lot of studies lately concerning the correlation between modern technologies and health. I read about one in the *New York Times* that said that, because of all of the numbers we are forced to remember for cell phones, fax machines, pagers, e-mail addresses, and bank PIN codes, to name a few, memory just cancels itself out. You remember the numbers, but you can't remember what you had for breakfast or what you wore two days ago. This made me wonder, has growing technology created a new niche in the medical arena?

Certainly. I consider myself a media ecologist. I have a great interest in studying the ways the innumerable waves of radiation—from computer screens, telecommunication satellites, radios, microwaves, and televisions—affect us physically, psychically, and intellectually. Modern medicine barely recognizes that they have any effect at all, but I believe the effect is huge.

Watch Your Water

Use filtered water. The water in most large cities is polluted. Purchase a filter that eliminates parasites, chlorine, and fluoride. Use a filter on your shower as well, especially if you are sensitive to chlorine.

Exercise Daily

Try a combination of yoga, body sculpting, interval aerobic training, and long walks in nature. Exercise both brain hemispheres: the left with reading and rigorous thinking; the right with music, art, and pattern recognition.

Meditate

Allow for periods of stilling the mind. Ask for guidance and remain confident that the answers will come. Practice using your intuition. When you make a decision, be sure it "feels" right. If it doesn't, don't do it.

Some say that living in this sea of waves actually enhances our intuition and makes us more sensitive to subtle energy. We become more affected by the right side of the brain, which is responsible for creativity and intuition. For women, who are naturally right-brain dominant, this further enhances our "sixth sense." For men, it awakens a part of them that is usually less dominant. The combined effect is that the electronic and digital environment could be making a great contribution to the merging and equality of the sexes.

I also think that as we are becoming more sensitized to the subtle energies that surround us, we become more aware of the energy in our own bodies and, consequently, more comfortable with and aware of the effectiveness of energy medicines like acupuncture, yoga, visualization, homeopathy, and herbs.

This trend toward accepting alternative medicine is not likely to lessen as the planet is miniaturized because of our digital environment. We are witnessing the amazing ability of technology to bring the whole world together. We have greater and greater access to other cultures, which allows us greater access to their ancient forms of medicine. We can share all of the many stories of people using age-old remedies with great success. It gives me hope and faith in humanity to see that people are so open to these various healing modalities. It's further evidence of the way in which technology is helping the world become a healthier global community.

Talk

I feed my soul by having long conversations with my spouse of 33 years and interacting with friends and strangers. I look for, and usually find, the divine in everything.

Save the Environment

Don't compromise on environmental issues. Don't allow pesticides and herbicides to be sprayed on you, your children, your home, or your lawn. Remind everyone that it is very inefficient to continue to use toxic products that create health problems in the population. Women's survival depends on the survival of the environment and our children. Since women are the main consumers in our society, we can vote with our pocketbooks by purchasing environmentally safe products.

WE ARE BECOMING MORE SENSITIVE TO THE SUBTLETIES OF EARTH AND MORE AWARE OF THE ENERGY IN OUR OWN BODIES.

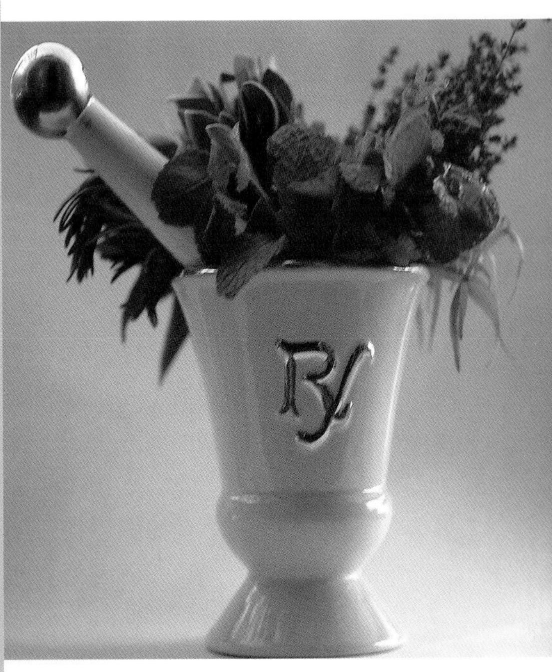

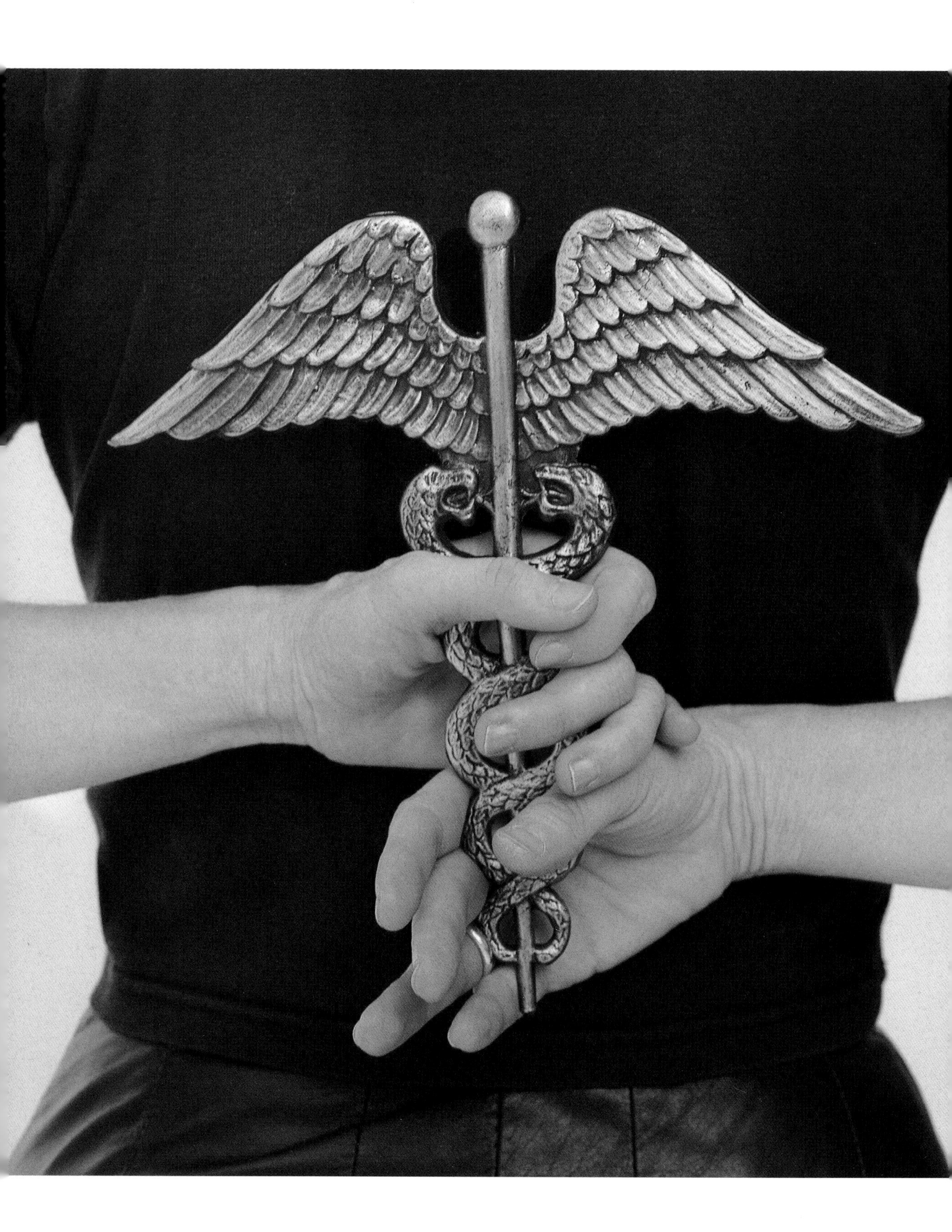

FIGHTING CANCER

Unfortunately, cancer will strike one in three women. I therefore think it is vitally important to offer the following resources to prevent cancer, which I am including in the upcoming new edition of my book, *Complementary Natural Prescriptions.*

AVOID KNOWN CANCER-CAUSING SOURCES

- Do not smoke or tolerate smoking in your family's presence.
- Avoid excessive exposure to sunlight and ultraviolet rays.
- Do not consider breast implants.
- Do not use dark hair dyes. Check out safe alternatives.
- Avoid perfumes, air-fresheners, perfumed deodorants, and antiperspirants containing benzene, aluminum, lemon-scented chemicals, and so on.
- Treat all cosmetic products with extreme suspicion until you have proof positive that they contain no known carcinogens. Safe alternatives exist, such as Aubrey Organics.
- Avoid dry-cleaned clothes. Find a nonchemical cleaner.
- Avoid chlorinated water. Use a water filter.
- Do not drink fluoridated water or use fluoridated toothpaste.
- Avoid electromagnetic fields (EMUs), especially with children. Use appropriate protection on your computer screen. Avoid living near hydro-towers. Avoid using a microwave oven. Keep cell phones away from your ear.
- Do not use hormone-disrupting or -mimicking substances such as chemical pesticides, herbicides, fertilizers, fungicides, and bug killers.
- Do not use cleaning, polishing, and renovation materials in your home that list unspecified "inert" ingredients or have toxic warning symbols.
- Reduce consumption of salt-cured, smoked, and nitrate-cured foods.
- Do not use meat or dairy products from animals routinely treated with antibiotics and raised with hormones or given bovine growth hormones to enhance milk production.
- Never heat shrinkwrapped foods or food in plastic containers. The plastic molecules—or xenobiotics—migrate into the food when heated.
- Avoid food additives, especially Red Dye No. 3, found in many junk foods and drinks. Avoid emulsifiers such as carrageenin. Do not consume hydrogenated vegetable oils or margarine.
- Do not drink or eat foods that contain sugar substitutes such as aspartame (NutraSweet and Equal). These contain wood alcohol, which can break down to formaldehyde in the body. Avoid refined sugar, which usually contains silicon. Stevia, unpasteurized honey-maple syrup, and brown rice syrup are healthy substitutes and easily available.
- If a doctor prescribes antibiotics, make sure that he or she has done the necessary test to identify the exact bacteria this antibiotic kills (except in extreme emergencies, like meningitis). Learn about natural alternatives.
- If a doctor prescribes prescription drugs, make sure he or she also gives you a copy of the drug's side effects and explains this information to you. If the drug requires regular liver function tests, ask your doctor to discuss the alternatives with you.
- Explore the alternatives to birth control pills, antihypertensives, antidepressants, hormone replacement therapy in pill form, and Tamoxifen as a preventive treatment. Get the full data on those drugs on the internet at www.preventcancer.com.

DO SOMETHING CONSTRUCTIVE ABOUT CANCER

- Have mercury amalgams removed by a dentist trained in the proper protocol.
- If overweight, have hormone levels checked and find out if you have food allergies. Overexposure to estrogen, lack of progesterone, thyroid problems brought on by pesticide exposure, or an adaptation to allergenic foods (wheat products and refined sugar) are frequent causes of obesity, which promotes cancer through excessive estrogen and pesticide storage.
- Exercise regularly and moderately.
- Eat cruciferous vegetables (like cauliflower, brussels sprouts, and broccoli), preferably organic. If that doesn't fit your budget, wash all your fruits and vegetables in VegiWash. This removes up to 97 percent of pesticide surface residues.
- Buy your foods in glass containers. Avoid cans and plastic.
- Take natural supplements. Avoid synthetics made from coal tar. Take charge of your health. If you need hormones, consider primarily natural ones and/or transdermally administered varieties in the smallest possible doses—they bypass the liver.
- Join a health or cancer activist group.
- Start a pesticide education group in your neighborhood. Read the *Journal of Pesticide Reform* for basic information. Subscribe to *A Friend Indeed* for reliable information on menopause and hormone issues (514-843-5730). Read Steingraber's *Living Downstream* (1999). Read R. N. Proctor's *Cancer Wars* (1995). Don't go shopping without *Dr. Epstein's Safe Shopper's Bible* (1999) or *Additive Alert* (1999). Read the classic by Adelle Davis, *Let's Get Well*. Read Dr. Epstein's *The Breast Cancer Prevention Program* (1999) and give it to your daughters, women friends, and others.
- If you have been recently diagnosed with cancer, search the web and other literature for effective options and choices. Your doctor is no doubt sincere but may not have studied anything but drugs, surgery, and radiation for cancer.
- Thoughtfully consider but carefully doubt all information (including this list) and start your own search for answers.

KATHY SMITH

Nationally recognized as America's fitness expert, Kathy Smith **has improved the quality of life** of millions of people around the world through her message of health and fitness. For more than twenty years she has made fitness accessible to people of all ages and fitness levels through her books, videos, national television appearances, and published columns. A dedicated mother, wife, entrepreneur, health and fitness expert, author, inventor, and television personality, Kathy Smith is an inspiration who will move us healthfully into the next century.

Q *The Century* by Peter Jennings and Todd Brewster is a collection of historically significant events that took place in the twentieth century, and your emergence as a fitness instructor twenty-five years ago was among them. How did you come to promote fitness as an integral part of life at a time when daily exercise was reserved for movie stars and professional athletes?

I was raised as a military brat. Every three years my family moved to a new base. I had an adventurous spirit but not a lot of security. When I was a senior in high school, my father—an air force pilot and outdoors man—dropped dead of a heart attack at the age of forty-two. It was a complete shock, and my whole world was instantly turned upside down. My mom, who had been a social drinker before my dad died, started drinking more and more. She remarried when I was a junior in college, but six months later she and her husband died in a plane crash.

All this happened between 1969 and 1973, a time characterized by the Vietnam War, the Kent State riots, the burning of the ROTC buildings, free love and drugs, and other anti-establishment activities. My parents were gone, and I was surrounded by chaos, upheaval, and questioning—at an age when a person already questions authority. It was a very confusing time for me. I was depressed and anxious, not knowing which way to turn and asking myself, "What difference does it make if I get a college education? Life could be taken away tomorrow."

In the middle of all this, I had a boyfriend who was a football player. He would go running in the off season and, in my quest to get close to him and because of my adventurous spirit, I started running with him on the track. Eventually I noticed that I felt clearer and calmer after a run. That's what first prompted my interest in fitness. I wanted to find out what it is about exercise that affects the mind so dramatically.

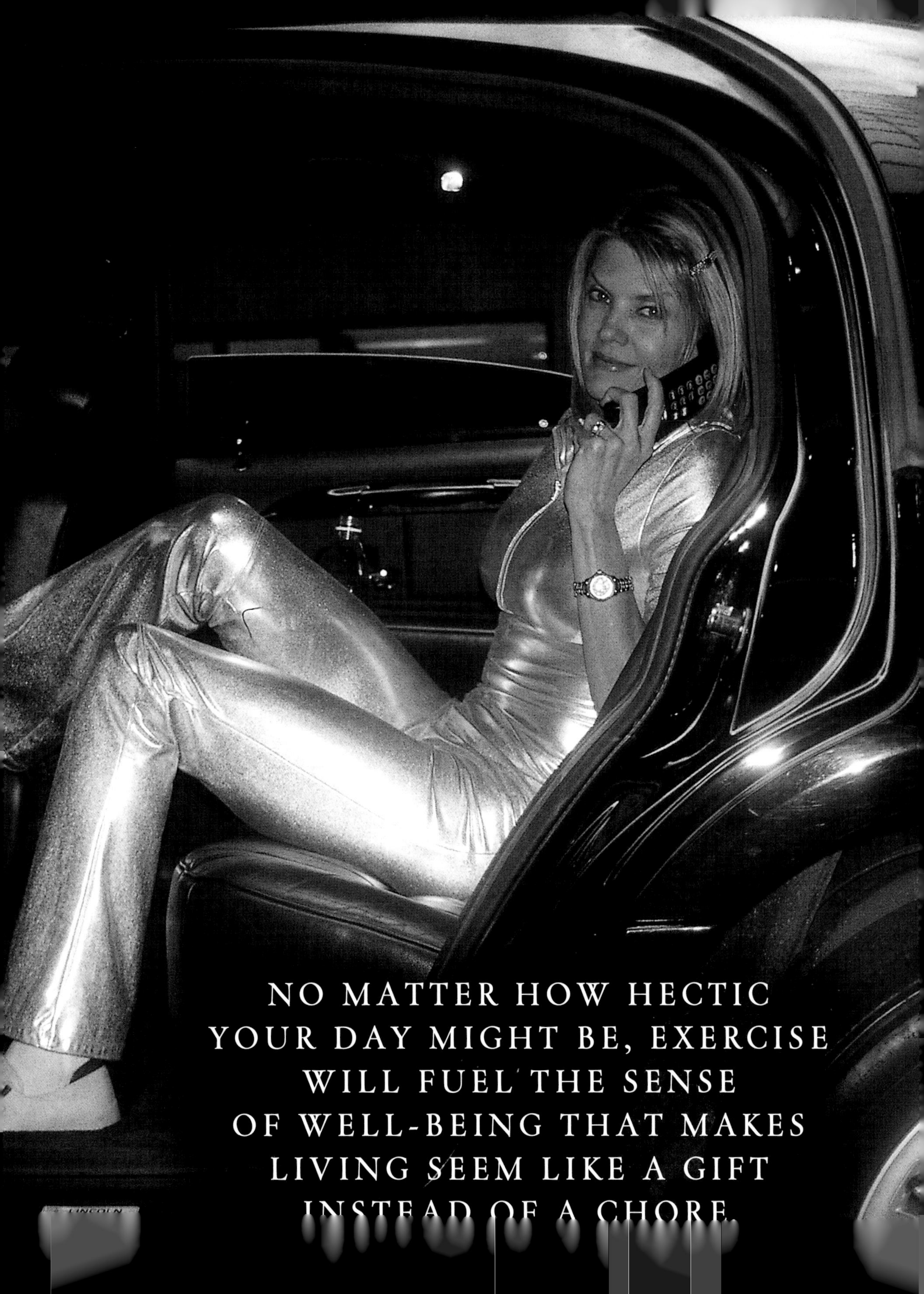
NO MATTER HOW HECTIC
YOUR DAY MIGHT BE, EXERCISE
WILL FUEL THE SENSE
OF WELL-BEING THAT MAKES
LIVING SEEM LIKE A GIFT
INSTEAD OF A CHORE.

What factors in your life turned your curiosity into an empire?

I became involved in long-distance and marathon running. I completed my first marathon in Hawaii in 1975, when there were not a lot of women in the running world. I loved the way I felt after I ran, but I also loved the brotherhood and sisterhood—the community of runners. I wanted to learn more about fitness, nutrition, and how the body works.

When I was in Los Angeles in the late seventies I started taking an exercise class. The only type available was the old-style calisthenics with arm circles and leg lifts taught by Gilda Marks. Barbra Streisand and Jane Fonda were also in that class. I loved the format of the classes and exercising to music, but I missed the aerobic component. So I decided to combine my dance background with what I learned about business in college and start my own exercise class. I quickly developed a following of women, and it was fascinating to hear how exercise changed their lives. This was pre–Title IX, before women were accepted into sports, so many of the women had never really moved their bodies like that before. For the first time, these women began taking care of themselves, which seemed to empower them to make other changes in their lives. The group became really tight-knit. They would come to class saying that they finally had the confidence to go get that job or that their sex life was better. That was very rewarding for me.

It seems as though you filled a void in women's lives at just the right time. I understand that your first product, a fitness record, went platinum.

Yes, and soon enough, someone asked me to be an instructor on a television show on USA network called *Alive and Well.* I was later asked to be a cohost for the show. We became the number-one daytime show for USA in the early eighties. I was also offered a book deal from Bantam.

In hindsight, I think about how easy it was for me. I was in the right place at the right time. But if you're handed an opportunity, it's so important to know if you can pull it off or if you're not prepared. I had moments of such self-doubt. Some days I would come home crying, thinking I was terrible. With almost no experience, I had been thrown into this job and was interviewing people on TV. So I did my homework. I got support in areas where I thought I needed to improve. I took voice classes and commercial classes. Before I made my first appearance on the *Merv Griffin Show*, my voice coach gave a bit of advice that I will always remember. He said, "Be yourself and be human." I remember being behind those curtains and saying quietly, "Be yourself." That was a huge growth point in my life, just learning to accept who I am. Aerobics and running also gave me confidence. If I had to leave my house at 5:30 A.M. to do the show, I would get up at 4:30 A.M. so I could run for an hour. I knew if I could get that run in, my confidence level would be high.

The show was two hours daily that first year, and I was nominated for an Ace award for best cohost on a cable TV show. I think that came from the fact that I loved what I did. It was about giving, helping, and motivating.

The idea that exercise is not only important for the body but also the brain is often overlooked. Body image is such a huge issue for women. What are your thoughts about women pursuing ideals that the media is pushing as opposed to just being healthy?

I think everyone should be the best and the healthiest they can be. They should focus on the really important things like their energy level and their mental state, and try to stay away from appearance. But there is no denying that people do care about how they look. And unfortunately, Hollywood tends to use only one body type, so most celebrities are leaner and longer-limbed. Women have to learn to accept that their bodies look and function differently than everyone else's.

It takes experience and some maturity to stop relying on the media to tell you how you should feel about your body. The problem is that the vast

Simplify

Exercise should be easy. The less complicated you make it, the more likely you are to do it on a consistent basis. So invest in a couple pairs of dumbbells and a treadmill and exercise while you watch the morning news. Recruit a neighbor or your spouse to walk with you three times a week after work. Join a gym that's within five minutes of your house and work out on your way to or from work.

Make It Fun

Exercise isn't limited to step-aerobics and running. And it certainly isn't something you have to do in a gym. Why not set up a regular tennis date with your spouse or a friend? Or go in-line skating or bicycle riding with your kids. Head to the local park and take your dog for a walk. Any activity that brings a smile to your face is one that's worth doing

Keep It Up

Nothing about exercise is harder than trying to start up from a dead stop. In fact, lack of energy is the number-one excuse people give for not exercising regularly. But it's a downward cycle: If you don't exercise, you can't be fit, and if you're not fit, you won't have the energy to exercise.

majority of Americans are still struggling with the simplest concept of a healthy life and how to feel good about themselves. It has to be a lifestyle. It starts with what goes into your body and extends into every aspect of how you live your life.

The most important question women should ask themselves is, "Do I take the time to exercise? Do I take a few moments to do something that will make me feel good about myself?" That's a great way to stop obsessing about whether or not your body is perfect. Just get out there and do something that makes you feel great.

Kathy Smith's FOCUS ON FITNESS

Consistency. Not perfection. We begin our new fitness programs with boundless energy and enthusiasm, intending never to miss a day of exercise or eat a morsel of fatty food. And while it's noble to aspire to perfection, it's unrealistic to think that anyone could be perfect all the time. After all, each of us is subject to emotional and physical highs and lows that impact our energy and commitment. But when they do, there's no need to throw in the towel on a healthy lifestyle. Better to do what you can when you can than to do nothing at all. If you accept the fact that, as Mama said, there'd be days like this, you'll be more likely not to abandon your program, no matter how many setbacks you think you've suffered. By walking a little when you can't run a lot, you make exercise a part of your life's fabric.

CONSISTENCY

Be passionate. I once read a fascinating report on longevity in which a researcher who had studied one hundred people in their nineties or older said he could find only two traits common to all of his subjects. The first: they had eaten a consistent diet their whole lives and had never experienced either extreme weight losses or gains. The second: they were all extremely interested in something outside of themselves—religion, a hobby, volunteering, and so on. Each of them, in other words, displayed a passion for something.

Even though it's my job, I still feel passionate about exercise—in fact, I revel in it. And I've learned that feeling vitally connected to one thing usually leads to other strong connections. My passion for exercise makes me passionate about life itself.

Whether or not our goal is to live past ninety, we owe it to ourselves to make the most of the time we're allotted here. Use your passion as a springboard. Find a fitness activity that puts a twinkle in your eyes and makes you feel like a child again.

DE-STRESS

De-stress your life. Here's the absolute truth: the number-one reason I exercise is because it gives me energy and helps me manage stress. Even if you are generally fit, you still have to watch for what I call energy "vamps"—as in vampires, those creatures that suck the life out of you. Always ready to drain you of strength, energy vamps come in different guises: lack of sleep, overtraining, undertraining, overeating, undereating, eating too much sugar, unexpressed anger, overexpressed anger, or relentless frustration. We must avoid our own energy vamps.

Change your mind-set. For years I've begun each morning the same way. As soon as I realize I'm awake—which is sometimes even before my eyes open—I start to focus on my breathing, taking long, deep breaths and listening to the sound of air rushing through my nostrils. I lie in bed for a few moments and make a mental list of what I'm grateful for. I'm a big believer in positive thinking; I believe that positive attracts positive, in terms of both moods and events. Without taking the time to number a few blessings, it's too easy to move right from sleep into the quicksand of panic or anxiety. This early-morning reflection is my way warding off the chatter that can be all-consuming in our society.

WORK IT OUT

Make exercise a priority. Here's one thing I've learned in my twenty years as a fitness professional: people who exercise on a regular basis don't have more time or fewer problems than anyone else. They've simply made exercise a habit—like brushing their teeth.

Stop thinking of exercise as that thing over there that you'll do when everything else on the to-do list gets done. You need to put it in the nonnegotiable category with brushing your teeth, tying your shoes, or even going to work. Some days you're really excited about getting to the office, and some days you're not. But you still go. Rarely do I open my eyes in the morning and shout, "Goody, I get to exercise today!" Like you, I often feel achy, or lazy, or depressed, or overwhelmed by crisis. But when those sensations plague me, I don't ask myself whether or not I should exercise. I get up, brush my teeth, tie my shoes—and exercise.

KEEP IT UP!

FOCUS ON FITNESS: DAILY ROUTINE

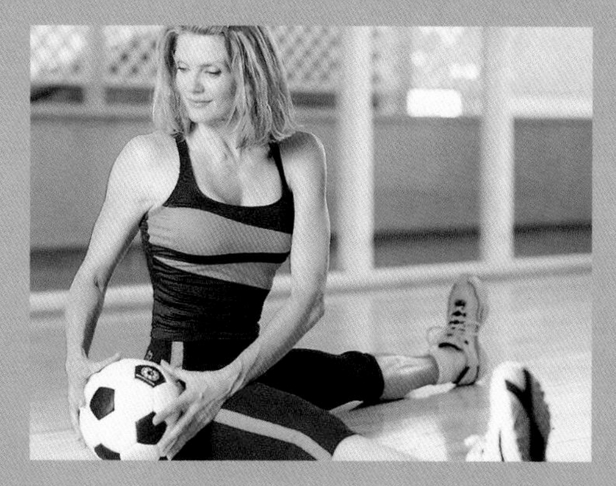

1. SEATED TWIST

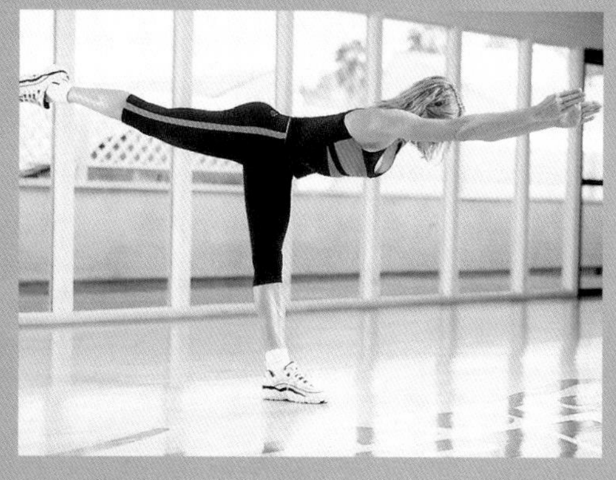

2. STANDING BALANCE POSE

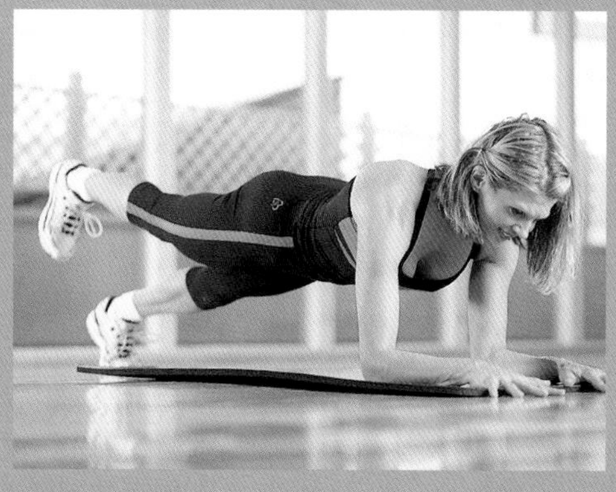

3. BENT-ARM PLANK

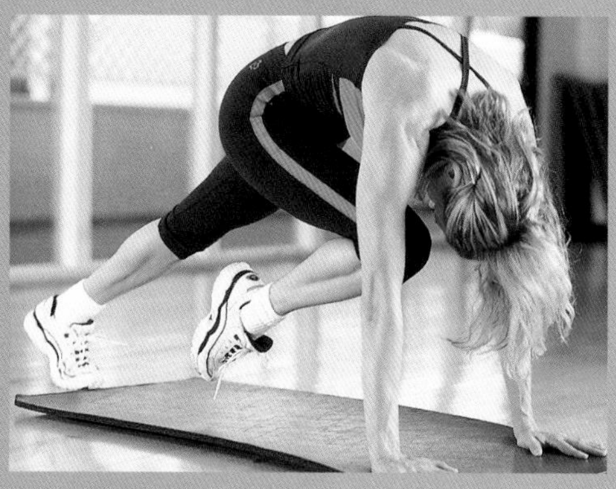

4. STRAIGHT-ARM PLANK

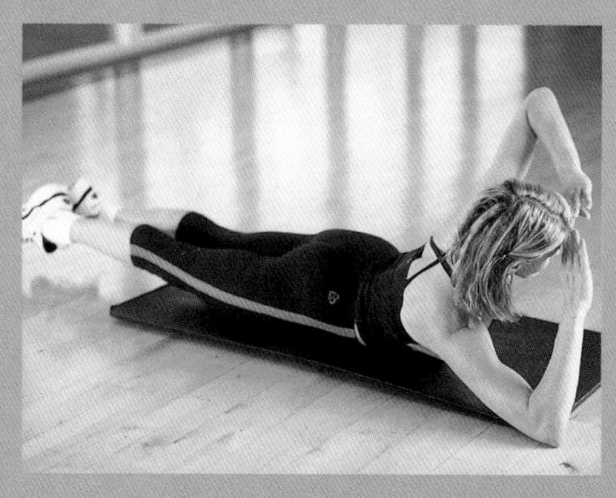

5. LOWER BACK EXTENSION WITH A TWIST

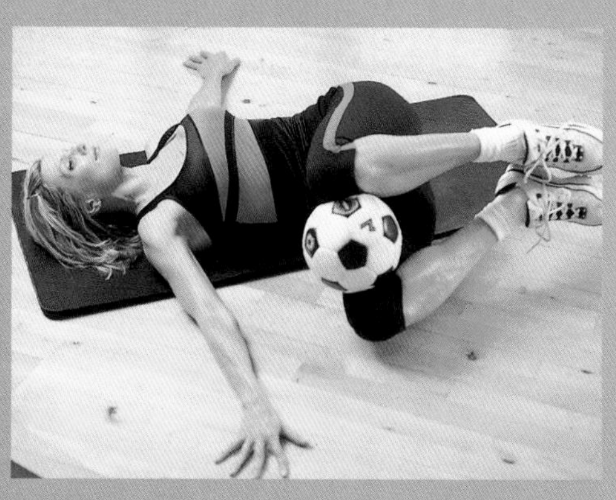

6. LYING HIP ROTATION

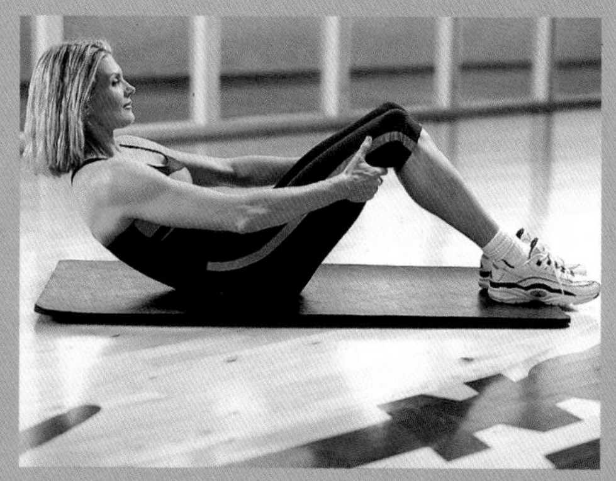

7. REVERSE ROLL DOWN

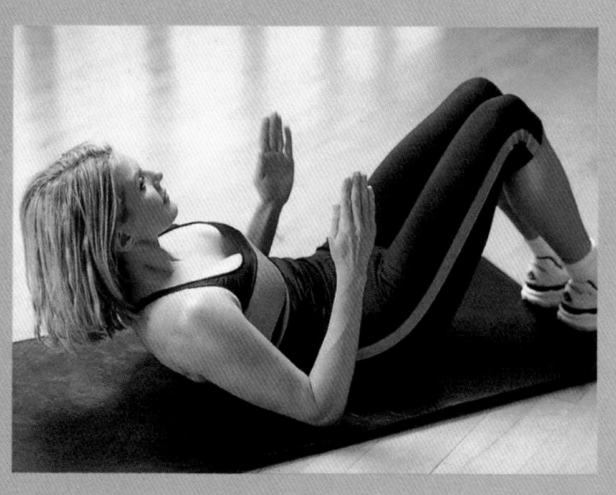

8. ASSISTED ABDOMINAL CRUNCH

Core Strength Workout

Strong arms and legs may look good, but the real source of strength in the human body is in your "core"–the muscles in the center of your body, an area that is comprised of your abdominal muscles and your back. Core exercises work the back and abdominal muscles that stabilize your torso. These exercises go beyond just strengthening your back and abs; they teach them how to work together to create a firm foundation. The only place your abdominal muscles work all by themselves is on the exercise mat–in real life every move you make involves this yin and yang of front and back. Core exercises duplicate movements that you actually make in real life, and what could be more effective than something you can actually use? Sit-ups do a great job of isolating your abdominals, but that's not the way your abdominals were meant to be used. The primary function of the abdominal muscles is to stabilize the spine in an upright position, not to fold in on themselves over and over. Everyone wants a flat stomach, but building washboard abs without strengthening your back at the same time can actually cause an imbalance.

1. SEATED TWIST Sit on the mat with legs extended in front of you in a V, with toes up and chest high. Hold a ball or 3- to 8-pound dumbbell in both hands. Sitting tall, slowly rotate torso to the right and place ball on the ground next to your hip. Contract abs and squeeze shoulder blades together as you sit up straight. Twist around to the other side and place the ball next to your left hip. Repeat all sets in a controlled manner.

Tip: Open legs wide enough to feel a stretch in your inner thighs and contract quads to stabilize your torso.

2. STANDING BALANCE POSE Stand tall with hands on waist. Contract abs and glutes. Shift weight to left leg and bend right leg so foot rests near left knee. Lift ribs to elongate spine, then contract your butt and slowly begin bending forward from your hips. Extend right leg straight behind, parallel to floor, as you reach out with both arms. Hold position for 10 seconds. (If lower back hurts, bend over to only 45 degrees.) Slowly come back to start. Alternate sides for consecutive sets.

Tip: Contract quadriceps muscle of your standing leg as you lower and raise your body, but be sure not to lock standing knee.

3. BENT-ARM PLANK Lie abs-down on the mat, supporting the upper body on your elbows (forearms are on the mat), toes on the floor. Contract glutes, chest, arms, and abs, and slowly raise your body in a straight line until only forearms and toes touch the floor. Raise right leg one to two feet off the floor. Hold for five to ten seconds, pulling abdominals, then lower your body down to the floor (drop leg and hips first). Repeat, alternating legs each time.

Tip: As you hold, focus on using chest and midback muscles to stay elevated.

4. STRAIGHT-ARM PLANK Lie abs-down, toes on floor and palms under shoulders in push-up position. Contract chest and arm muscles as you slowly press your body up in a straight line until palms and toes touch floor and arms are straight (don't lock elbows). Tighten abs and glutes and lift right knee slowly into chest; tuck chin in slightly. Hold here for five seconds, then return right foot to floor. Alternate sides.

Tip: As you bring knee into chest, round back slightly and contract triceps and shoulders to stabilize the move.

5. LOWER BACK EXTENSION WITH A TWIST Lie abs-down on mat, toes on floor. Place hands against your forehead or on the back of your head, elbows out to sides. Contract abs and glutes hard and slowly lift right shoulder and chest off mat (keep left elbow on floor). Twist up and back through the right side of torso until right elbow points up to the ceiling. Keep head still and chin down to avoid straining neck. Hold for five seconds, then slowly switch sides.

Tip: Keep hips on floor--flex butt muscles as you raise and lower.

6. LYING HIP ROTATION Lie back on the mat with arms extended at your sides. Bend knees 90 degrees but keep feet a few inches off the floor. Place a big ball (use a folded pillow if you don't have a ball) between knees and slowly rotate at the waist, dropping your legs to the left. Touch left knee to floor, hold briefly, then bring legs back to center and repeat on other side. Keep abs tight, palms down, and shoulder blades and midback glued to the floor at all times.

Tip: As you roll legs to each side, contract your abs hard and tighten your obliques (the muscles around your waistline).

7. REVERSE ROLL DOWN Sit up super-straight with knees bent, feet flat on floor, and hands grasping the backs of your thighs. With abs taut, slowly begin lowering your back to the floor. Just when you reach the midpoint—shoulder blades are about six inches from the mat—cross arms over chest and take five more seconds to sink the rest of the way down; sit up and repeat. (Beginners may want to start off with one or two sets instead of three.)

Tip: Contract arms and chest as you lower upper body to the floor.

8. ASSISTED ABDOMINAL CRUNCH Lie back on mat with knees bent and feet flat. Place elbows at your sides, point fingertips to ceiling, and press lower back firmly to mat. Crunch up slowly until shoulder blades clear the floor, and press elbows into the mat to lift yourself higher. Keeping upper arms stationary, hold up for five seconds, then lower and repeat.

Tip: Visualize your rib cage moving closer to your hips as you lift higher and contract your shoulder muscles.

Every day I relearn life by watching my two-year-old son. He goes about his day in a flow of freedom. Free from self-consciousness, connected to his deepest intuition, and eager to gain as much knowledge as possible. As we grow older we tend to lose that enthusiasm; we become homogenized, intellectualized, socialized, and eventually set in our ways. Our overwhelming rationality prevents us from expanding our minds toward new intelligence—emotional and creative as well as practical.

In order to open our minds to new possibilities we must lose our fear of being wrong. This can be a daunting task for women because many of us have overcompensated and fought so hard to be heard. I myself am guilty of this. I can think of many instances when my gender has played against me but none as significant as my experience in graduate school. While working toward my master's degree I had the misfortune of encountering a series of very biased instructors. One in particular insisted

nd

on never calling me by my correct name, choosing names like Cindy and Bambi, and would often pass over me at round-table discussions. In case you were wondering, that instructor was a woman. On another occasion, a film I made was viewed by a prominent film critic during a visit to the school. It was a very serious film about the tragic death of my grandfather as told by his two daughters. The critic gave it a rave review and even cited it as an example of the perfect sibling movie. The instructor's only comment was "Yeah, sometimes you can create art that is so inane it's almost brilliant." This, along with several other negative incidents, stayed with me for years, crippling my ability to find the deeper meaning of my life, and drove me toward closed-mindedness. I became overwhelmed with the pursuit of perfection, believing that if I had perfect accomplishments, no one could question me.

A lot of women experience this pressure to prove themselves, whether it's running a company or baking a cake. Throughout our lives we need to remember to think freely, break out of habitual responses, and be open to new lessons. We can live fully and magically in every minute, and work on self-improvement without fear of rejection. Only when we overcome our fear of being wrong can we truly harness the power of our minds. Ellen McGirt is the perfect example of this type of renewed independence. She teaches us that women can overcome our love/hate relationship with money and use our intuition to become financially successful. Cynthia Rowley declares that living artfully is all about being oneself and enjoying all things in life–even the not-so-perfect. All the women featured in this section share jewels of emotional intelligence, creativity, and clarity of mind.

DR. CHRISTIANE NORTHRUP

Dr. Christiane Northrup's **vision of mind-body wellness** has received an extraordinary response from women all over the world. Her award-winning book, *Women's Bodies, Women's Wisdom*, powerfully demonstrates that when women change the basic conditions of their lives that lead to health problems, they heal faster, more completely, and with far fewer medical interventions. Trained at Dartmouth Medical School and Tufts New England Medical Center, Northrup cofounded the Women to Women Health Care Center in Yarmouth, Maine, which has become a model for women's clinics nationwide.

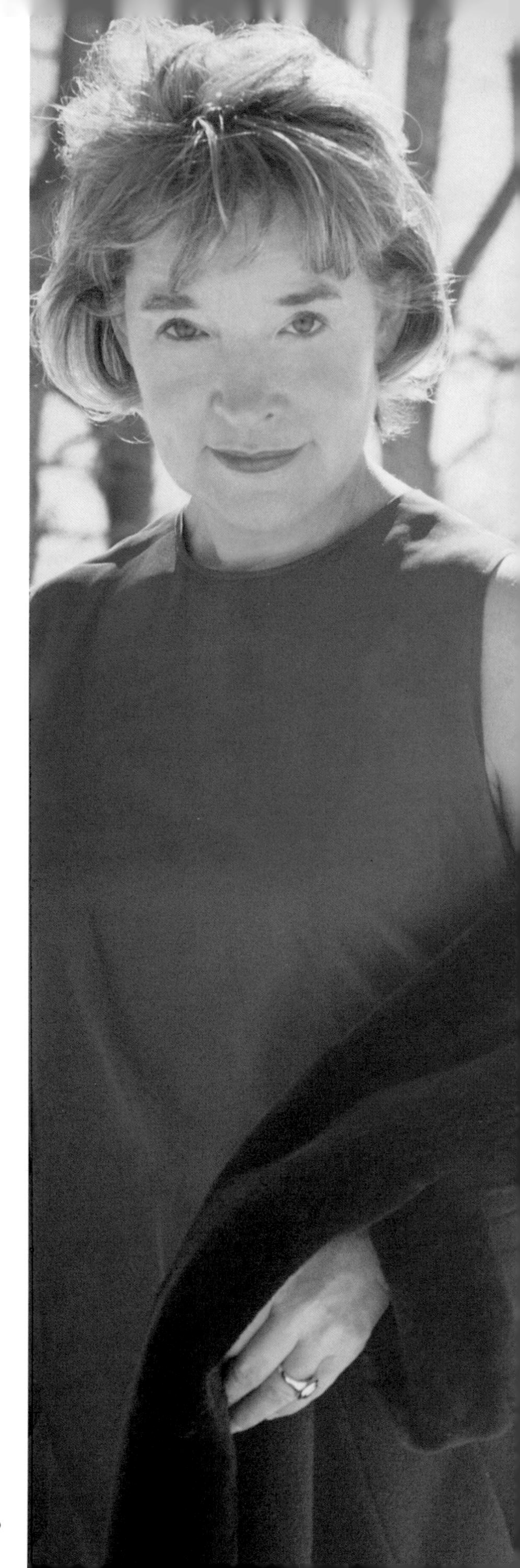

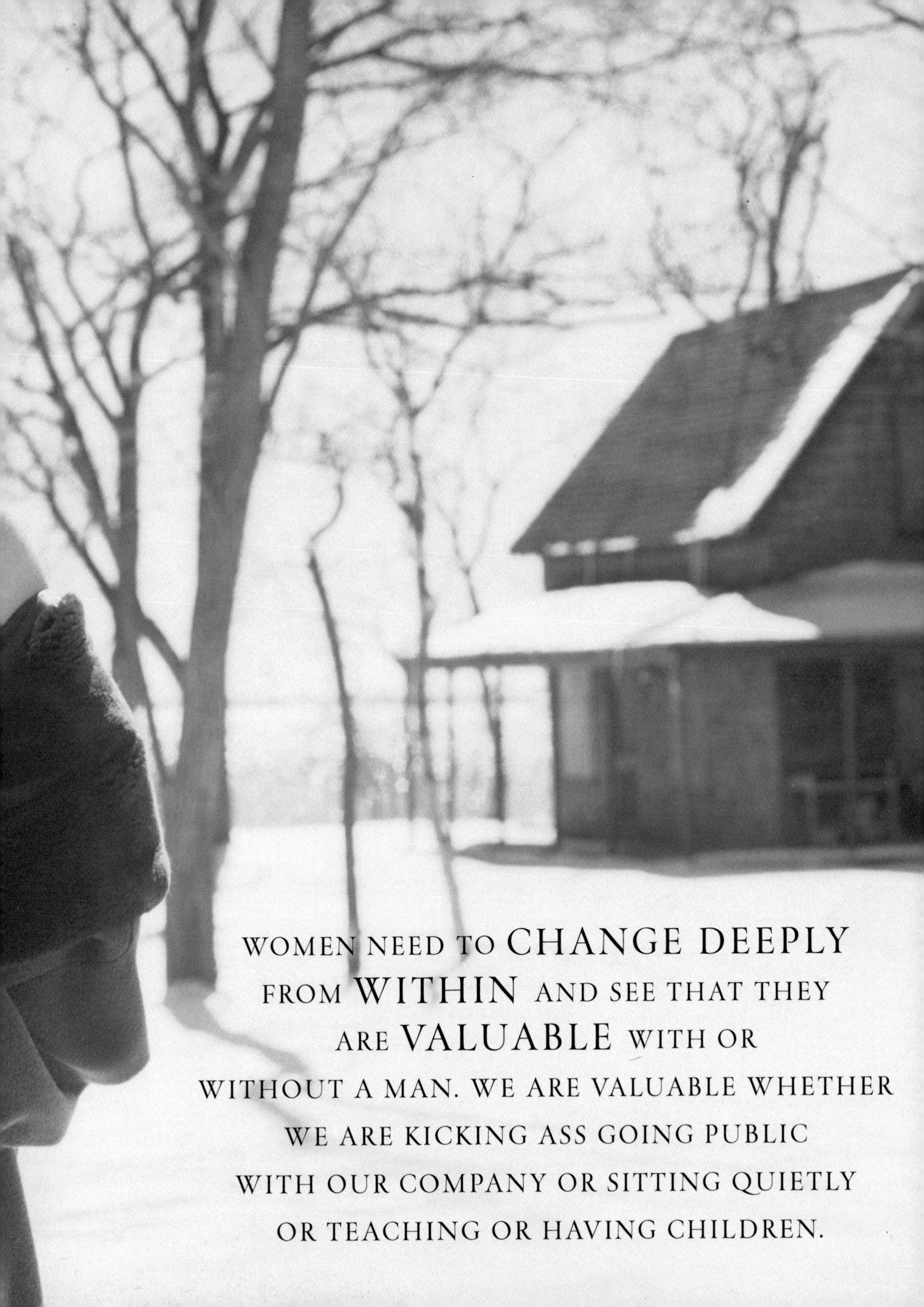
WOMEN NEED TO CHANGE DEEPLY
FROM WITHIN AND SEE THAT THEY
ARE VALUABLE WITH OR
WITHOUT A MAN. WE ARE VALUABLE WHETHER
WE ARE KICKING ASS GOING PUBLIC
WITH OUR COMPANY OR SITTING QUIETLY
OR TEACHING OR HAVING CHILDREN.

Q How have women's everyday problems changed in recent years? Does the working woman have a new set of concerns?

It's really the same doll, different dress. The only thing that has changed is that people are more educated, more savvy than they have ever been. And the number of choices available for staying healthy has made it more confusing than the old patriarchal system of "I'm the doctor. Do what I say." In some ways that old way works better. The doctor says do this, and you do it, and everything is fine, and you don't have to worry about it or keep a copy of your charts. Some people are scared by the freedom of choice; I see more confusion now.

Because of this, my primary aim these days is to teach people to find the solution within them. I have a huge practice through my newsletter, and the most frequent question I am asked is "How can I find someone like you where I am?" The truth is, people usually don't need to do a lot with a doctor. They need to change their thinking patterns. Then it's just a matter of going for a visit now and again when you can't figure it out yourself. We are consumed with thinking we need to see doctors.

We need to look at illnesses as wake-up calls, even if they are painful. They bring us back to our body and ground us. It's an obvious solution but it seems that people need to hear it from an authoritative position. I think that that's the reason I became an MD, so I could validate what people already know.

Q Can you talk about the patriarchal myth and addictive system you refer to in your book?

The patriarchal system is an internalized belief that that which is male is better than that which is female. And when I say that, I am not talking just about men versus women as gender. I'm talking about a way of being in the world. It's the thought that we must cut to the chase, get to the point, summarize, be quicker, bigger, better, more. For example, I was meeting with a law firm recently about doing more web stuff. They speak about a "hundred-day plan" and how the venture capitalists are on you, so you need a "kick-ass CEO." That is very testosterone-based thinking. Women have plenty of testosterone, and it really kicks in at midlife, and I'm all for that. But I know that we also must honor the feminine part of us in service to our soul and in service to a higher vision. The higher vision is not about going public in two years and retiring to the beach because then what are you going to do? You are still left with an empty soul.

And here's an example of the power we invest in the patriarchal system that really gets me because I see a whole new generation of young women buying into it. My sixteen-year-old daughter is living in a cabin on the coast of Maine for a semester with eight guys and twenty-four girls. There is a core group of young women who do nothing but hang around the guys. They're all intensely well educated and still they believe that their value is determined by male attention.

The movie *American Beauty* has a wonderful scene in which the Annette Bening character begins to have an emotion and wants to cry. But instead, she yells at herself to stop. That's the patriarchal myth–a woman's sadness, emotions, need for rest, nourishment, and a fulfilling spiritual existence are not good enough. Those needs and expressions are not considered to be critically valuable. During the women's movement back in the seventies women liked to think that they would be empowered if the culture changed. And while that is part of it–I got into medical school very easily because it was the time of the woman–we're not going to change anything until women change deeply from within and see that they are valuable with or without a man. We are valuable whether we are kicking ass and going public with our company or if we are crying and shouting or if we are sitting quietly or if we are teaching or having children.

Get Out

Get outside regularly. The sunlight and air have amazing healing properties. With all of our climate-controlled buildings and artificial lights, it's more important than ever to get some natural light. It is a great way to enhance your immune system.

Breathe

Breathe fully. Many women are shallow breathers who only use the upper one-third of their lungs. By exercising your diaphragm, you trigger the parasympathetic nervous system—the rest-and-restore system—calming down the sympathetic nervous system's fight-or-flight hormones.

Positive Focus

Take five minutes to notice the things that are working in your life. Write them down. Make this a habit. Going back and reflecting on the positive versus the negative will increase the body's ability to avoid and combat illness. Avoid things that make you anxious; don't watch the news if it makes you feel scared or upset.

Q With technology changing so quickly, the competition to keep up is really powerful. It's so easy to get wrapped up in that and forget to take a moment to step back and look at what you're doing and how you're doing it.

Yes, keeping up is a really powerful draw. Whenever I am tempted to sign one of those stupid contracts and sell my soul and dance with the devil—and believe me, I have had lots of offers recently to do just that—I am always brought back to what I have been seeing from the time I began my training in the seventies. What do I see over and over that destroys a person's health? It is the constant sense that someone is going to beat you to the top. I have seen enough people at the top to know that that does not create health or happiness. You can't earn enough money to get healthy or fill your soul. On the other hand, you can't get sick enough to make someone else happy or healthy either. That's another place I see women going. They want to save the world by getting into social work or digging ditches in Somalia. That doesn't do it either. The only thing that does it is to tune in to what brings the most joy to your life. Find those things that make you cry when you are premenstrual or perimenopausal—those activities or thoughts in which you lose yourself to a bigger picture. One way for people to have that experience is to go to rock concerts or sporting events. We key into large group activities that make us part of something bigger than ourselves and that, ultimately, is very nourishing.

Q Society and the medical world say that stress is the cause of many of our problems. But they fail to clarify what stress. What do you say to people who attribute their problems to life's stress and things outside of their control?

I once wrote a newsletter article called "The Myth of Stress." We use the term *stress* to hide behind rather than doing the hard work of changing the specific conditions of our lives that lead to this amorphous biochemical state that is connected with ill health. There are two extreme groups of people when it comes to dealing with the stress of life. One group meditates when they feel stress. So they don't get anything accomplished because they are over in the corner saying, "Ohm." The second group of people are completely addicted to stress. They tend to work in places like emergency rooms or in investment banking.

Then there are people somewhere in the middle who have the courage to say to their spouses or children, "When you say 'x' I don't like it and it bothers me in a very specific way." That's when you have identified the stress that negatively affects your health and are dealing with it.

Most people will use the phrase "I'm stressed" as a socially approved way to avoid taking responsibility for the next step in their lives. Each of us has to look at the way in which we, in particular, are living this mindset. What affects people most of all is how they think and how they behave in the microcosm of their own lives. These are the things that have the most power to create or destroy our health.

Doctors are as guilty of enabling that as any other group, particularly with women. In OB/GYN, which is my specialty, they have been quite good about bringing to the attention of us practitioners the prevalence of domestic violence; it's the number-one cause of premature death in women. It's a perfect example of how our culture has to evolve, because women are giving more than we're getting. Perhaps it's because of the patriarchal myth or because our brothers were more respected than we were or because if a girl has any ambition and acts out one-third as much as a boy in grade school, she is seen as a behavioral problem (he's just being a boy). We're sure that we're not as valuable as the male, so he preys on this.

Q Could you tell me the basic principles women should follow when they are thinking about things that are affecting their health.

Take this on faith until you see the evidence of it in your own life: 99.9 percent of biochemistry moves toward health at all times. You can't will your blood pH to stay where it is; it just does it. When you breathe in, you oxygenate the hemoglobin in your red blood cells. When you cut yourself, you heal. What we need to do is focus more on what is working in our bodies and in our lives every single day. Despite artificial light and moving through time zones and all the rest of the things we do to compromise our well-being, our periods still come once a month. It's an unbelievable miracle, biologically speaking.

We are tuned in enough to the moon that our periods come once a month regardless of almost anything we do. That's the most important principle: look for evidence of well-being in your body every day. I think our culture has become overzealous in looking for what's wrong. The mantra is to be afraid of your next Pap smear, breast exam, or mammogram, but women need to keep giving themselves evidence of what is working. It's a change in mind-set, but if you do it all the time, you will see how well you are and how well you can keep yourself. It will help you tune in to the subtle changes in your body. And if you can recognize them early on, you may, with a small amount of effort, be able to keep yourself well.

Q What new issues have concerned you since you wrote *Women's Bodies, Women's Wisdom*?

I'm currently working on a book about the wisdom of menopause and the developmental stage that women enter during menopause. There is a chapter about menopause in *Women's Bodies, Women's Wisdom*, but I wrote it before I went through the change myself. I was forty-eight then and well into premenopause, but my periods hadn't really stopped yet. They have now that I'm fifty, and I can see that, at this stage, the brain also changes. You begin to think differently. Your worldview changes. You get down to your essence, and that's pretty exciting.

Even after having seen hundreds of women go through menopause, I didn't get what it was about until I went through it myself. I have always tried to see the deepest meaning behind the biological processes of the feminine body, and I can only do that after I have been through them myself. Our culture likes to reduce the changes that women experience to raging hormonal events of all kinds, whether it's postpartum depression or PMS or menstrual cramps. Ours is a patriarchal culture; it only makes sense that women are made to feel shameful of the times they are most powerful. We are told that we are victims of our hormones, but I always knew that that was not how the creator set it up, that there had to be some deeper meaning. Once I started going through menopause, I started to say to myself, "Oh, I see. Just when I am really smart, really able to contribute, possibly at the height of everything—strength, sexuality, skill, intelligence—society conspires to make me feel washed up and over the hill." It's that kind of thinking that keeps the status quo for women.

Q What drives you to do what you do? And where do you see that taking you next?

I believe that my next path here is to learn something about changing our genetic inheritance. There's a way in which genes are expressed or not, depending on the environment in which they find themselves. People are feeling more powerless than ever because we have given them genetic reasons why they're going to get heart disease or breast cancer. Therefore, the need to balance this with transformative, empowering, actionable information is greater than ever. Right now, nothing excites me more than that.

I am realizing that what I wrote in *Women's Bodies, Women's Wisdom* is becoming more true for me the older I get: there is evidence of women's wisdom springing up all over the place, including in men. Identifying and encouraging this is a driving force inside me. I am constantly moved by the ability to listen within myself. I am thrilled each and every day that I have been able to tap into something as powerful as my feminine voice and I can't wait to find out where it leads me next and how I am going to share that with the rest of the world. The feminine voice is the voice of the soul and it comes through our bodies. It's always there asking for our attention. I am seeing that now more than ever. I feel it in myself and see it in other women. It is just so powerful and exciting. And we have just barely begun.

Respect Your Body

Respecting yourself will help you reach your optimal size. The feelings associated with self-respect create a metabolic milieu in your body that is conducive to optimal fat burning. By contrast, the metabolic processes associated with emotional stress tend to keep body fat firmly in place.

Eat Slowly

Eating small amounts of foods you crave, such as chocolate, balances the brain chemistry in women by increasing seitonin levels. If you don't allow yourself to indulge modestly in these cravings your desire for them will likely increase to uncontrollable levels. Savor them slowly and fully.

Eat Properly

By eating when hungry and stopping when full, you learn to tune in to your body's wisdom. Reassure yourself that you can eat when you are hungry and can stop when full, but not bursting. Try this: wait fifteen minutes when you still want a bit more. Fifteen minutes is about how long it takes for the brain to register fullness.

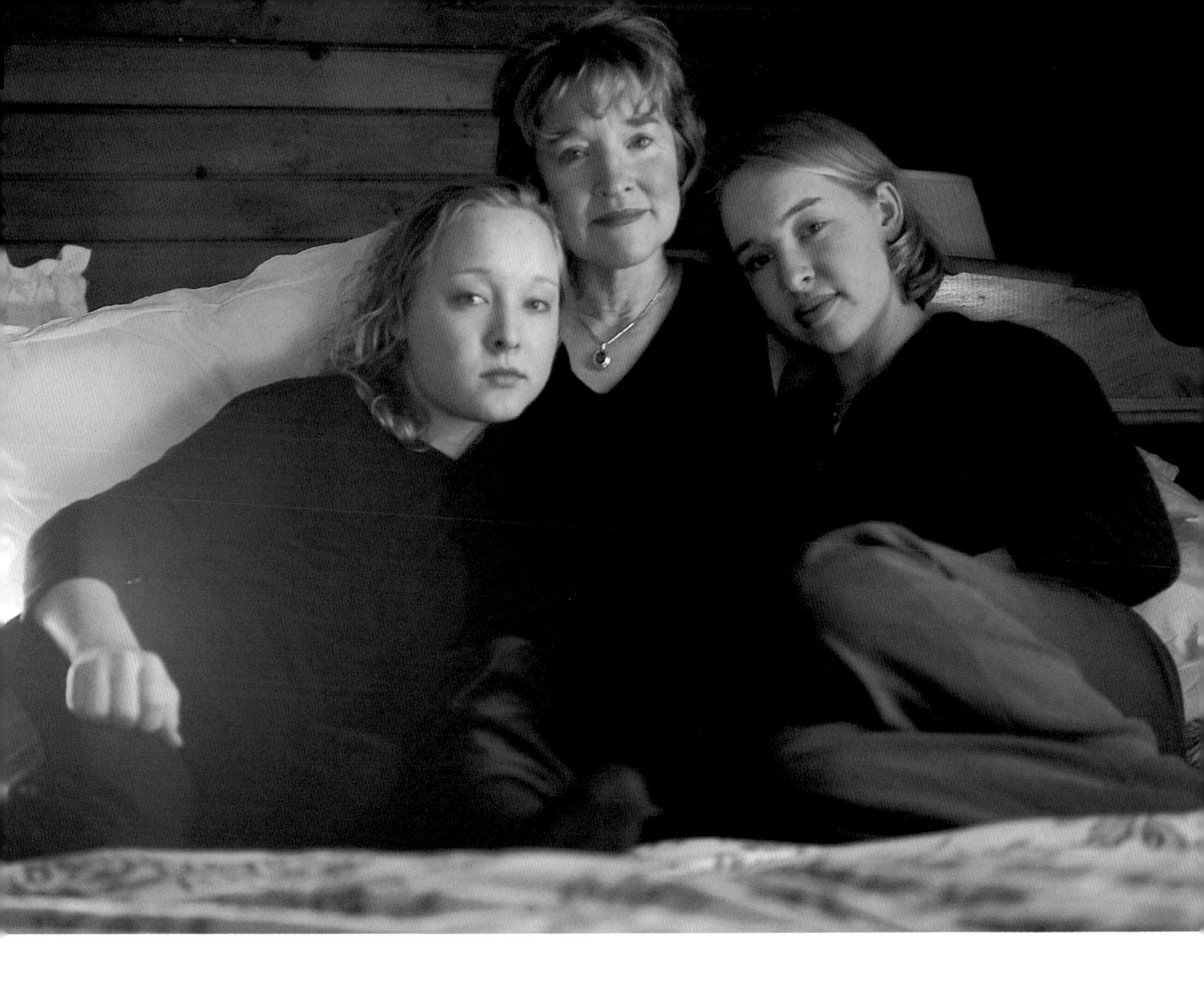

MOTHER-DAUGHTER WISDOM

Raising two daughters has provided me with uncompromising training for letting go and allowing someone else to grow, make her own decisions, and live her own life. I've known that I am not the higher power for either of my daughters from the time they were babies. At the same time, my job as their mother was to engender a deep sense of safety and security in each of them by giving them a nurturing space in which they could grow and evolve according to the dictates of their own souls. I like to think that my relationship with both of them is almost completely devoid of the negative side of family obligation, which includes dread, fatigue, and guilt that is often perpetuated from one generation to the next. My daughters are not symbols of me—their lives are entirely different. They are proud of me, and I am proud of them. They look forward to the future unafraid, each directed by a deep connection with her inner wisdom and a strong sense of self. I do the same.

The Power of Positivity

When women change the basic conditions of their lives that have led to health problems, they heal faster, more completely, and with far fewer medical interventions. The key to change lies in our ability to reconnect with our inner selves. We must not ignore our true needs and feelings. By doing so, we create the illusion that we can control our lives. The following six examples are characteristics that we have all used to separate ourselves from our emotions, forcing us to believe that it is possible to be completely objective and unemotional when it comes to our health. By reversing this train of thought, we release the power of positive thinking.

SYNDROME	DEFINITION	EXAMPLE
NEGATIVISM	Seeing life from a lackful viewpoint	"I always catch whatever is going around." "Now that I'm forty, everything is starting to fall apart." "You can't have that, it costs too much."
DEPENDENCY	Believing that someone or something outside of you will take care of you because you can't do it for yourself	"I can't leave my husband. Who would support me?" "I can't live without him."
CRISIS ORIENTATION	Using or creating an external crisis as a socially acceptable way to distract yourself from your feelings	"There's no question that we really look forward to the next multiple trauma. It gets the juices flowing." – Emergency-room nurse.
DEFENSIVENESS	Being unable to accept feedback and make positive adjustments	"Who are you to tell me that my PMS is related to my family? My childhood was perfect."
DISHONESTY	Not telling the truth	"Do I need a break? No, I'm fine." "It wasn't that bad. I can handle it."
DUALISTIC THINKING	Believing that there are only two choices: one is right or good, the other is wrong or bad	"Vitamins and herbs are good. Drugs and surgery are bad."

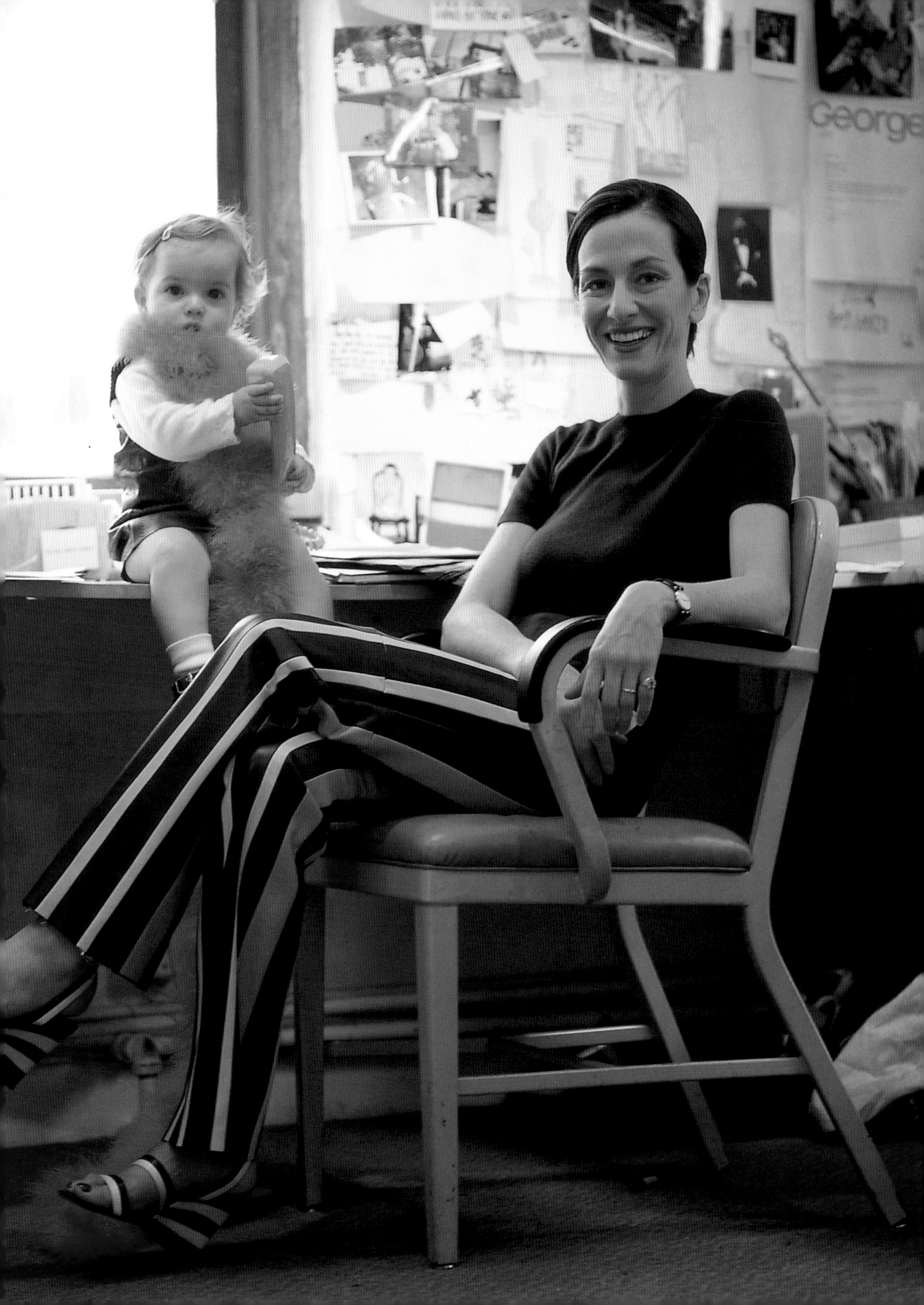

Q You're such an original designer—you never mold your style to meet the industry standard. I read that your mother was a big influence in your creative life.

I had a real white-picket-fence childhood in small-town Illinois. My mom was at home, and my dad was a science teacher, and dinner was on the table at 6:00. My childhood was a happy twinkly inspiration. It's so sappy. But the flip side was that there was nothing to do, so we would make stuff. My dad is like MacGyver, jerry-rigging everything. My mom was an artist. She came from a very creative family: her parents were painters and her brother is an art teacher and sculptor. When I grew up my mom didn't let us have coloring books because the lines were already there. I wanted a chatty Cathy doll but my mom said that I had to create my own conversations. It got a little wacky. We would even dress up for dinner on "theme night." Looking back now, I realize that that's where my creativity came from. But at the time, I just thought everyone's moms short-sheeted their beds for a laugh.

Q When did you get into fashion?

I always used to draw and sew, but it wasn't until I went to art school for college that I even heard of fashion designers. Barrington, Illinois, is like the golf-shirt, Talbot's capital of the world–nobody knew about Parisian or New York designers. But my roommate was very cosmopolitan and she showed me a Calvin Klein jeans ad with Brooke Shields and said, "He's a fashion designer–why don't you do that? It's like sewing and drawing combined."

Q Your sense of design is eclectic but very feminine. It has a little bit of class and a lot of whimsy. Did you plan to design for women specifically?

I never had a plan. I just was making stuff. I did not know there were factories that would make this stuff or that buyers buy certain things. I was so clueless. I once made a small collection with huge mohair sweaters and wool coats and some buyer said to me, "The whole world isn't like the Midwest. Other people don't have such harsh winters." It's still coming together for me every day. I often have realizations and think, "Oh, that's how you do it."

My only goal has been to continue to live an artful life in every sense of the word. I have never worked for anyone. I just do. It really comes from my mother and grandmother, who never said, "You can't." I want my own daughter to love life and experience and appreciate it fully. I never want her to feel locked into one way of seeing things.

Q Is that the advice you give women who come to you for fashion tips? In your book *Swell* you describe living artfully as living life with style and spirit—navigating life's curves with a little bit of swagger and a whole lot of grace.

Living artfully goes beyond fashion. Don't worry about breaking the rules. Just be yourself. What do you have to lose? It's the same in every part of your life. Just try it, work hard, be thankful. A lot of people think it's never good enough. They think what they have done or are doing is never enough, or that there is a right way of doing things.

Everything is so commercial today. There's too much pressure on women to be and look a certain way. They get this idea that if it's not perfect or it's not pricey it's no good. People want a sort of precious perfection. But perfection is overrated. It's much more important to be yourself. Enjoy all things in life, even the not-so-perfect. If you can't do it the highfalutin way, do it your own way. Do it for yourself. That is so much more real.

For example, we think that McDonald's is the second choice, but sometimes McDonald's is what you want. So have a party and serve that. Ilene and I had a dinner party and we didn't have time to make anything. So we ordered all the food the night of the party. We ordered steaks from one place and then we wondered where to get french fries for steak frites. And we thought of McDonald's–they have the best fries. We found out that McDonald's delivers and so we had the food delivered while everyone was there. We weren't shy about it, and that was the best part.

I do things like that every day. I paint our stores myself. And I love adding things to the collection that are really eclectic. I just finished a beautiful coat made from a vintage bedspread that I bought upstate. I once used curtains from an old house to make tapestry coats that were kind of faded and cool. People thought they were fabulous. The point is that living artfully isn't about spending money. It's about enjoying the simplicities of life and not misconstruing simple beauty and uncomplicated fun for mundane.

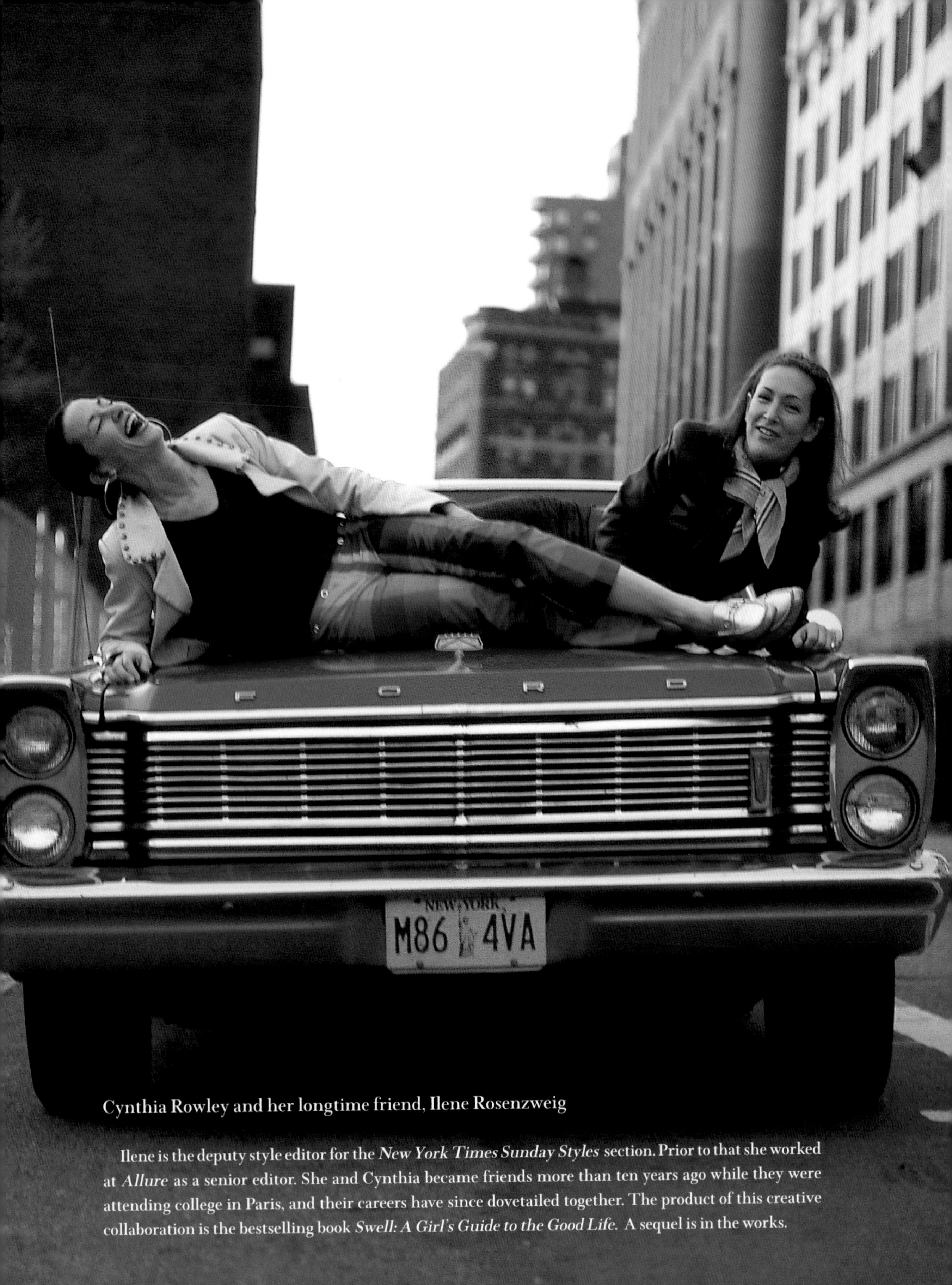

Cynthia Rowley and her longtime friend, Ilene Rosenzweig

Ilene is the deputy style editor for the *New York Times Sunday Styles* section. Prior to that she worked at *Allure* as a senior editor. She and Cynthia became friends more than ten years ago while they were attending college in Paris, and their careers have since dovetailed together. The product of this creative collaboration is the bestselling book *Swell: A Girl's Guide to the Good Life.* A sequel is in the works.

Top Tips for Girls

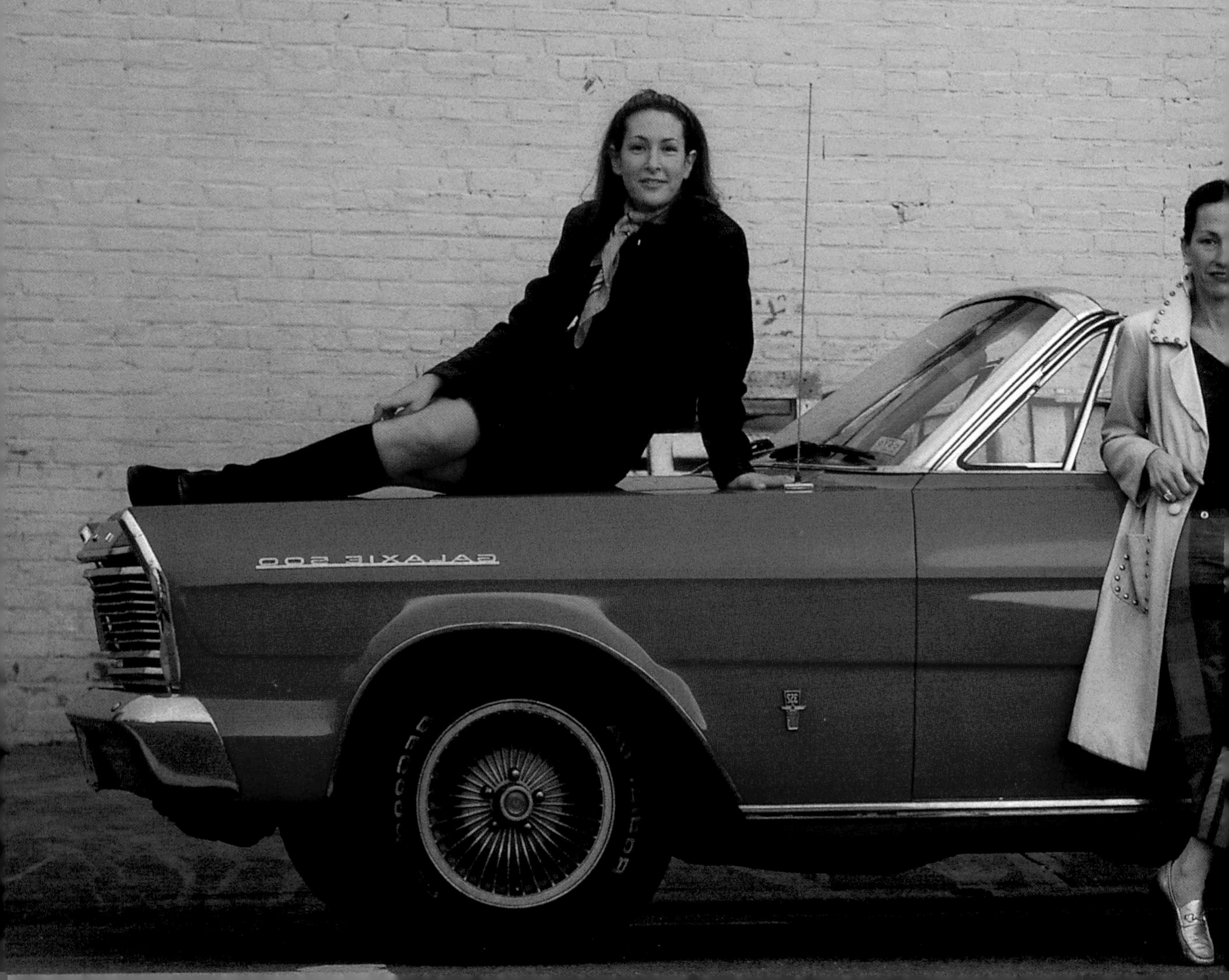

on the GO GO GO!

By Cynthia Rowley and Ilene Rosenzweig

OUR IDEA OF POLITE SOCIETY IS NOT WHERE TO PUT THE SOUP SPOONS...

The imperfect hostess. What she lacks in time and resources she makes up for with ingenuity, her speed dial, and the Pretty Good Housekeeping Seal of Approval.

Make big parties small. Whether it's a wedding for two hundred or dinner for two, keep it personal. Mix traditional with unconventional, formal with informal, caviar with deviled eggs. Follow your own tastes even if they don't seem to go together. Cynthia's wedding took place at an airplane hanger in Brooklyn with a DC3 as a centerpiece. Instead of separate tables, she used one long table with love poems written in marker on the tablecloth. Boarding cards with seat assignments were handed to guests. She wanted her guests to have their own cakes so cupcakes were arranged, each with its own bride and groom on top. Each personal touch made it even more romantic.

Make small parties big. Not everything has to be a production planned weeks in advance. The last-minute blast is all in the packaging. Lack of Irish linens is no excuse for avoiding having people for a sit-down dinner. Why get so serious? Try road maps with a globe as a centerpiece. Or just plain paper with the guests' names scrawled at their places. Napkin rings can be key chains, bow ties, and plastic watches. For an off-centerpiece, arrange a bouquet of framed baby pictures—each guest brings one and has to guess who's who.

Dinner for six. (You're leaving the office at five.) Here's the perfect menu: Whip through the grocery store like a supermarket sweepstakes contestant. Two chickens (nothing's simpler than roast chicken if someone else did the roasting), goat cheese logs, blueberries, a Sara Lee Cheesecake (you'll see), baby carrots, and newborn spuds (small things cook faster and look cuter). Hurl veggies into roasting pan, drizzle with olive oil, salt, and pepper, toss into oven. The clock is ticking. Roll cheese logs like Playdough into adorable heart shape, flatten, and sprinkle with chopped tomatoes and crushed crackers. Drop birds in with veggies to reheat (sprinkle them with rosemary to resuscitate). After successful meal, run back to kitchen, sit Sara Lee on plate, rinse berries, place in pan with teaspoon of sugar for brief time over low flame. Pour over cake, letting goo drip down sides (mess = homemade). For extra credit, split cheesecake horizontally by pulling a piece of dental floss through and add goop to middle layer. Voila!

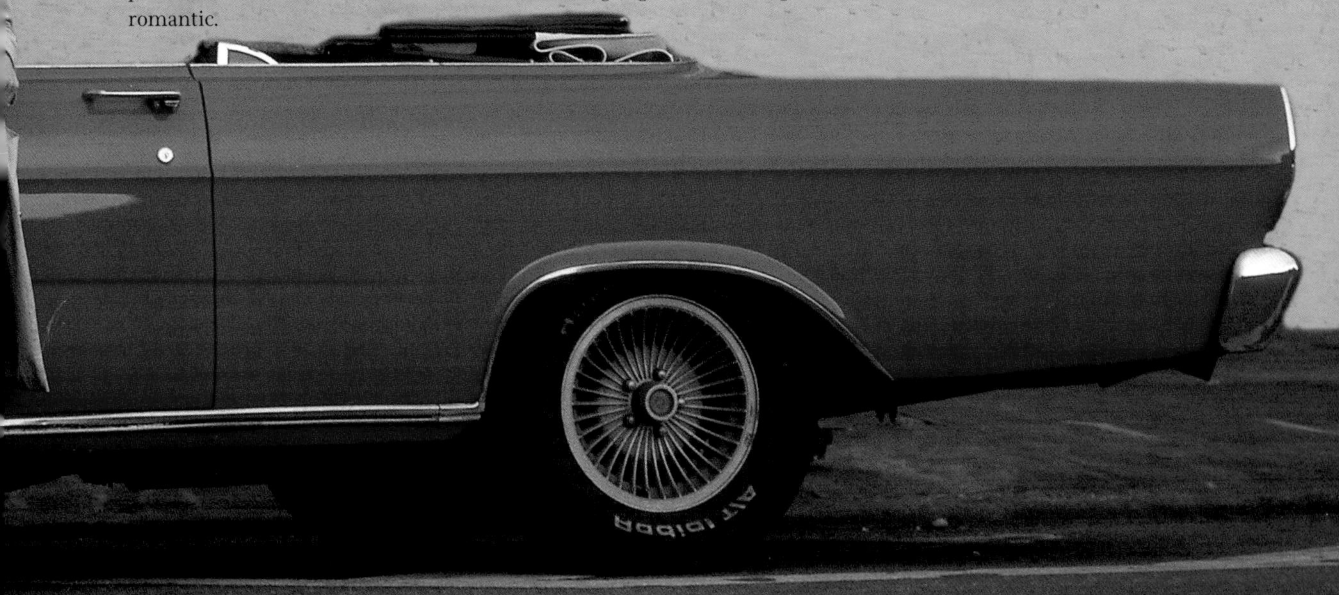

Top Tips for Girls on the GO GO GO!

continued

Love. Go ahead and take a gamble, so what if you lose your shirt? Love's a crapshoot—you don't always hit seven on the first roll. Keep in mind that a good gambler doesn't sweat every hand. Remember, not every affair ends up at the Elvis Chapel, but that doesn't mean that it wasn't worth the trip to Vegas.

Think of love as an action flick, not a five-hankie weeper. It's filled with chemical explosions, suspense, and, of course, great chase scenes. Whether he's on your tail or you're heading after him the wrong way down a one-way street, make scenes memorable, packed with bold responses, surprising twists, some innocent subterfuge, and spontaneous invitations.

The morning after. Scram, or scrambled eggs? If you wake up and realize that this is all a big mistake, set the clock ahead two hours and feign panic: "Oh my gosh, it's ten o'clock, I have to get to work." On the other hand, if you wake up and think you're still dreaming, figure out a way to make Sunday last all day long. Not by asking meekly, "What are you doing today?" (Puts him on the spot.) Tell him what you've got in store: "I'm going to the Museum of Television and Radio to watch some classic *Mission Impossible* episodes." If he looks interested, tell him to grab his hat because the invitation will self-destruct in five minutes.

The sweetie called at work to tell you he misses you and you bit his head off. Explain your stress quota all you want, but an explanation without contrition is just rationalization. "I'm stressed" is not an apology. "I'm sorry" is. Those two words cannot be overvalued. They don't cost a dime but they buy a lot of good will.

Whether you've been dating five days or married five years, you can always ask your heartthrob if he's free on Saturday night. The anti-date can be the antidote to relationship ennui. Skip the popcorn and porn—too obvious. Try another take: Japanese Horror Night. Serve cold sushi and hot sake. Slip in and out of your Kimono geisha-style. And when you cry "Oh Godzilla!" move your lips a few seconds before letting out sound.

Check into motel sex. When looking for the idyllic getaway, you don't have to drive five hours to Quaintsville, USA. Just pull off the interstate. There's nothing sexier than a motel room stocked with all the necessities for an illicit rendezvous. Magic fingers! Fifty-eight channels. Okay, so there are no mountains to hike. Naked relays to the ice machine burn calories, too.

Look pretty. Just because a girl's got a big caboose doesn't mean she can't be a looker. A great beauty cannot be measured by the sum of her anatomically correct parts. She's got to have that certain something. What that certain something is can be hard to pin down. It's all in there somewhere. Just tease it out.

Invisible makeup. At the gym, on a camping trip, there are times when wearing makeup makes a girl look like she's got something to hide. No one will detect these invisible tricks: add a touch of eyelash glue to the brows and brush with a toothbrush to hold them in the finished shape; line lips and fill in with neutral pencil, then coat with lip balm; apply a few dabs of blush before moisturizer.

Gravity-defying boobs. Going strapless or backless? Create the illusion of buoyancy with remarkably simple tape technology: one or two strips of electrical or masking adhesive that go from one armpit to the other, pressed beneath the breasts in the line where underwire would go, thus pushing them up and together. Caution: destickify tape on fabric before applying to skin so as not to remove boob when removing tape.

Cryogenics. An easy answer to awaken a dead complexion. Rub an ice cube over your face before applying makeup. Watch skin tighten and circulation increase in seconds. Marilu Henner and Joan Crawford's trick.

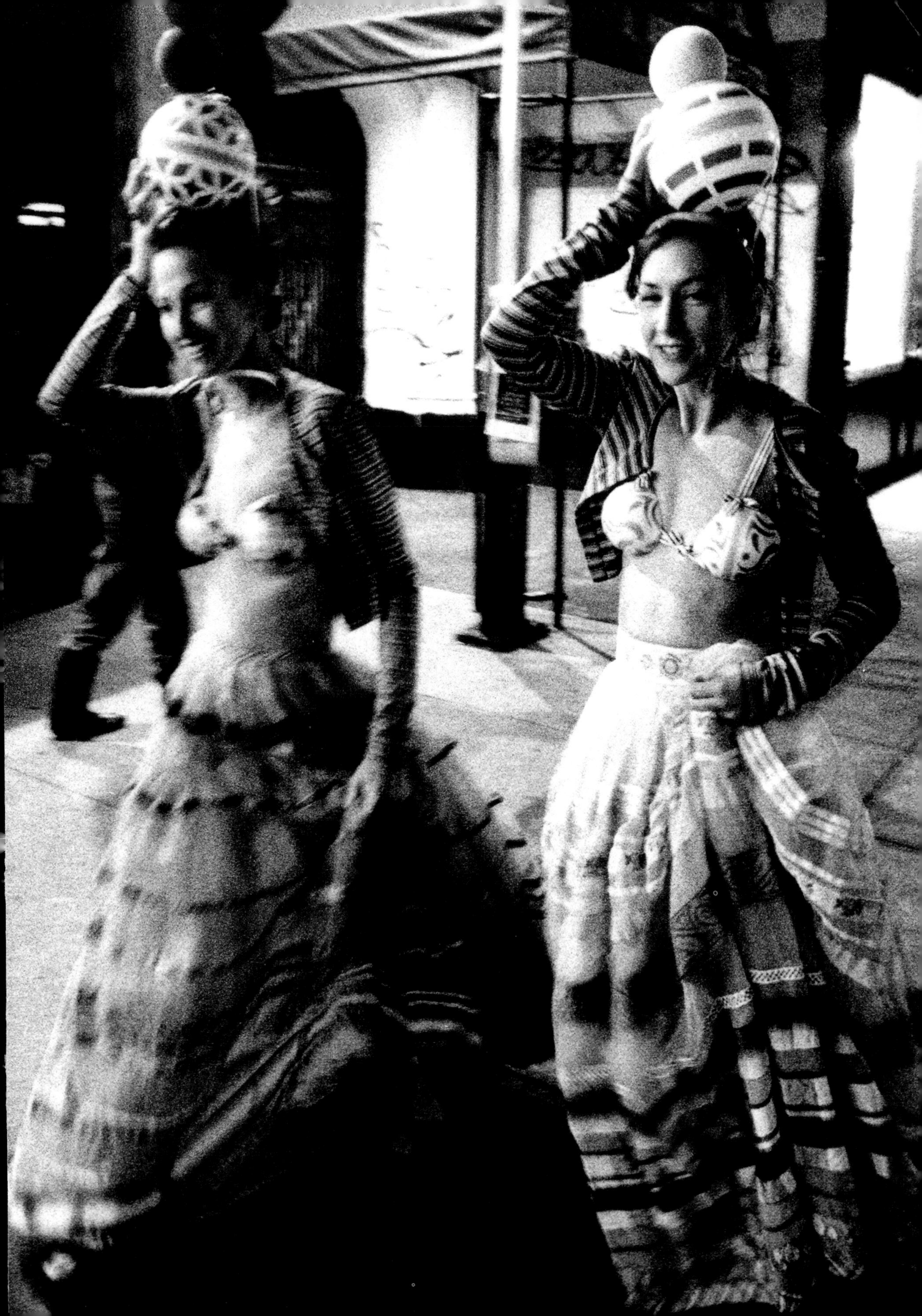

ELLEN McGIRT

Financial wizard Ellen McGirt **never imagined she would be giving investment tips to thousands of women each week.** She joined a brokerage firm midcareer in a desperate effort to gain financial insight. As a broker, she met remarkable women of all ages and backgrounds who sought financial independence and inspired her to write about her experience. Her first foray into financial writing was *Cassandra's Revenge*, an online guide to wealth, money, and happiness for women. Now, as the voice behind Oxygen Media's *ka-Ching*, she is able to take her training, experience, and insight to a wider audience.

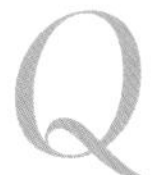

Seventy-five percent of elderly people living below the poverty line are women. How can we stop this cycle of financial ignorance?

Let's face it, ladies, the promised rose garden hosts some real thorns. Most of us will not get married as soon or stay married as long as we expect to, due to general busyness, divorce, or that annoying habit we have of living an average of seven to ten years longer than men. Whether we want to or not, nine out of ten of us will be on our own financially, managing our own money at some time in our lives.

According to the most recent census, nearly 65 percent of women between the ages of thirty-five and forty-four are part of the workforce. How easy do you think it is for them to work, climb the ladder, raise or hunt for a family, stay healthy, and still look good in spandex? (Come on, everyone wants to be attractive.)

On the other hand, the average woman will spend 14.7 years away from the workforce, while her male counterpart will spend an average of only 1.6 years away. This lost income and the lack of pension contributions and other investment opportunities result in a devastating effect on a woman's financial security.

Q **These are unsettling statistics. How can we motivate ourselves to change after thinking about all that we've missed out on in the past?**

Don't get mad, don't put your head in the sand—get even. Remember, success is the best revenge and the only acceptable attitude for a new and improved female investor. Besides, it's more fun. And if you're married, chances are your husband will be thrilled. It's something you can work on together.

The good news is that the limiting cultural stereotypes that keep us comfortable rather than wealthy can also work in our favor. Consider the following gender stereotypes and how natural our understanding of financial markets can be:

WOMEN AREN'T AFRAID TO ASK FOR DIRECTIONS. Good thing, because you'll need them. Forget those nasty exchanges over folded road maps while the gas station attendant looks blankly at your angry mate. You're driving now. Ask the experts for their favorite routes to wealth. Listen to their answers. Subscribe to newsletters (especially the free ones). Go to investment conferences. Read books. Hit the internet. Then, take your own road.

WOMEN UNDERSTAND CYCLES. Boy, do we ever. Throw in a little delayed gratification (nine months and you get . . . more work!) and you've got the perfect investment mind-set. Investment markets are cyclical. True wealth is created through long-term strategic planning. You've got it made.

One overpriced lunch, six lattes, and four movie rental late fees = $50.00 a month. **$50 a month, invested in an account returning an average of 10% (which is lower than the return of the overall market since 1926), will be worth $113,024 in 30 years.**

Today's woman of 62 has logged nearly 50% fewer years of paid work and has earned a 33% lower salary than a man of the same age. **Today's man of 62 can expect to receive four times the retirement benefits that his female counterpart will receive.**

Learn to embrace risk as an important tool in investing and in life.
If you fail to take sufficient risks, prepare to let life pass you by. Take too much of the wrong risk and prepare for a bumpy ride.

One unnecessary pair of shoes, two long-distance sympathy cell-phone calls, and an unused 10-class card at the gym = $150 a month. **$150 a month, invested in an account returning an average of 10%, will be worth $339,073 in 30 years.**

Women are not culturally prohibited from asking for directions. This is good, because we'll need them to navigate a rapidly changing and uncertain world. **Women consistently spend more on psychic hotlines, horoscopes, and other "magic" advice than we do on financial advice.**

Keep at least three months' worth of living expenses in a liquid account for emergencies. Make sure you are adequately insured. Know what's on your credit report and have your own credit card. Put all brokerage or banking complaints in writing. Check in with your advisors regularly. And don't screw around with the tax man. Ever.

Statistically, **male investors place trades on their accounts on the average of 45% more frequently than do female investors**, significantly lowering their overall returns. Women continue to earn on the average of 75 cents to every dollar earned by a man. Yet, we are responsible for over 80% of all purchases, inside and outside of the household.

Two parking tickets, one new toy du jour, six jumbo cookies, one guilt-laden, overpriced "sorry I forgot" gift, and two credit-card late fees = $300. **$300 a month, invested in an account returning an average of 10%, will be worth $678,146 in 30 years.**

Don't let the lifestyles of others dictate your money goals. Missing your kids' bedtime every night because you are struggling to keep up with the car lease is missing the point.

ANKA RADAKOVICH

Sex advice columnist **Anka Radakovich is a world-renowned author and television personality.** For nine years Anka wrote the wildly popular sex column for *Details* magazine. Her two books, *The Wild Girls Club* and *Sexplorations*, have been published in Germany, Japan, Australia, and the Czech Republic, as well as in the United States. She is currently at work on a new television series and a screenplay with Paramount Pictures.

Q **How did you become a sex columnist?**

I think my motivation at first was to entertain my readers, but after I had written a few columns, I realized that a part of me wanted to talk about my bad dates so that men would begin to treat women with more respect. When I go out on a first date with a guy, and he pushes my head down at the end of the night—that behavior just has to be made fun of! At first I thought that guys would get mad at me for making fun of them, but I started getting letters from guys thanking me for being frank about sexuality. Besides, they always seemed to think I was talking about some other jerk.

I have always found sexual behavior fascinating. And my parents were very open about sexuality; they thought that sexuality was a natural part of life and not something to get uptight about. I remember going to the store with my parents when I was twelve and feeling particularly self-conscious about my new "developments." My mother, who was an opera singer, started making jokes about her own big boobs and I thought she was cool for relieving my embarrassment. Then my father started commenting on some guy's eyes popping out as he leered at her boobs and I thought that was hilarious. I was sexually curious at an early age, and my mother answered all my questions. I was a bit surprised at the time, but now I'm glad she gave me all the facts instead of having to find out in the back seat of a car from a creepy pervert.

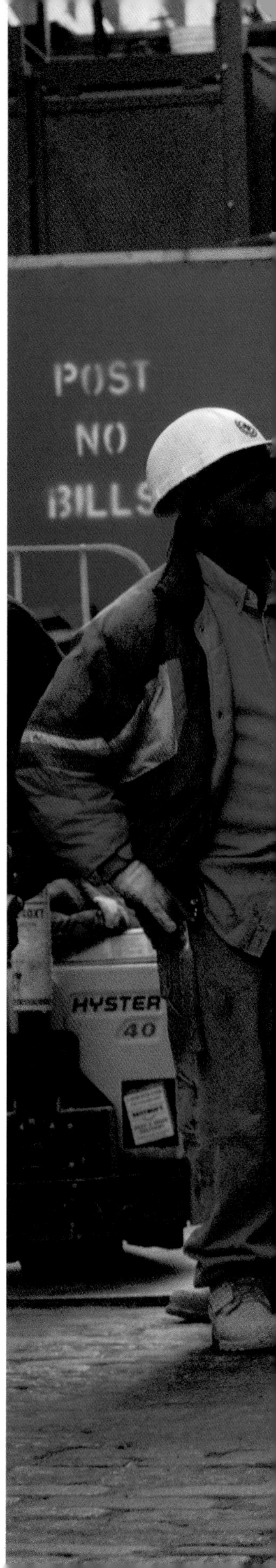

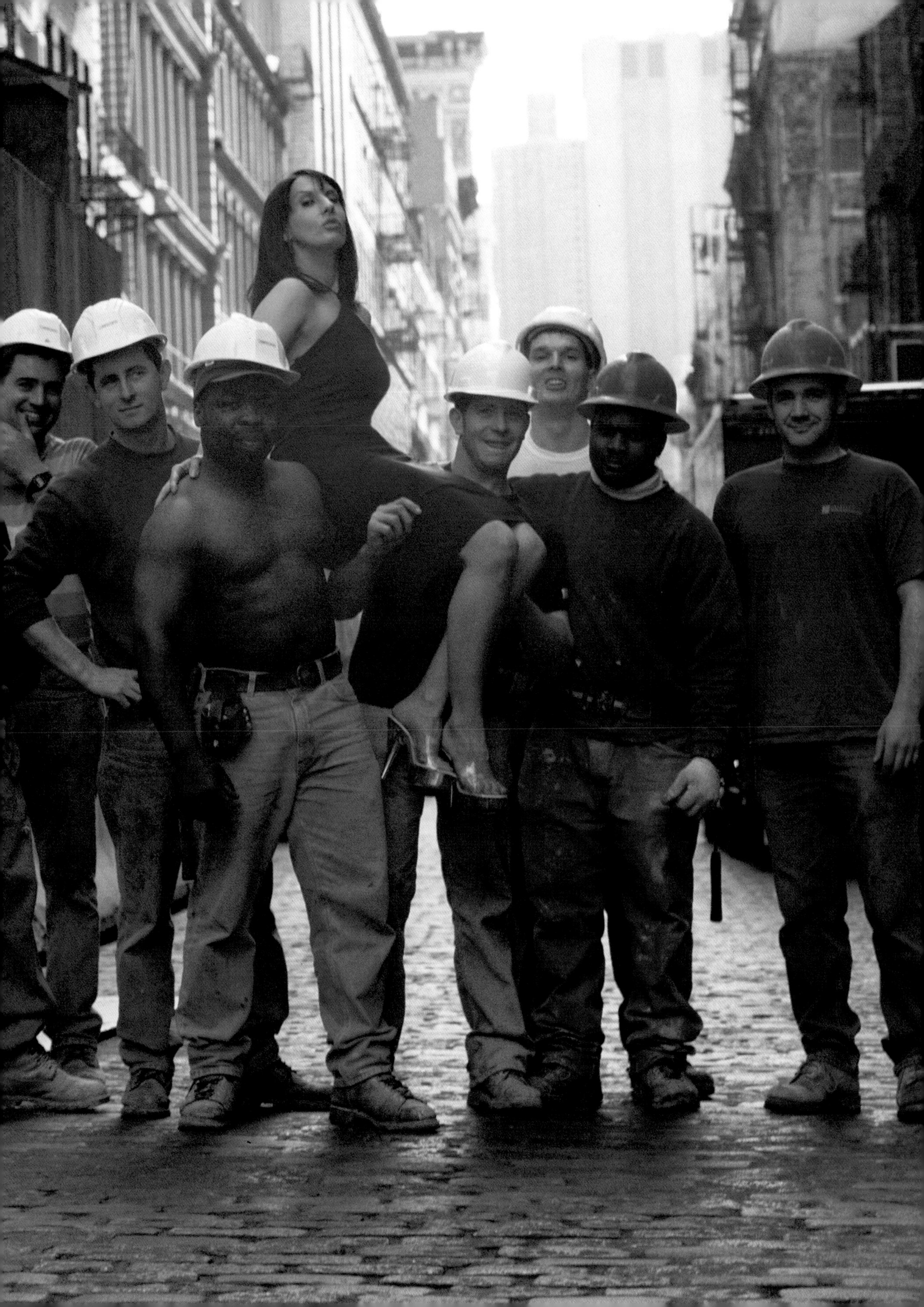

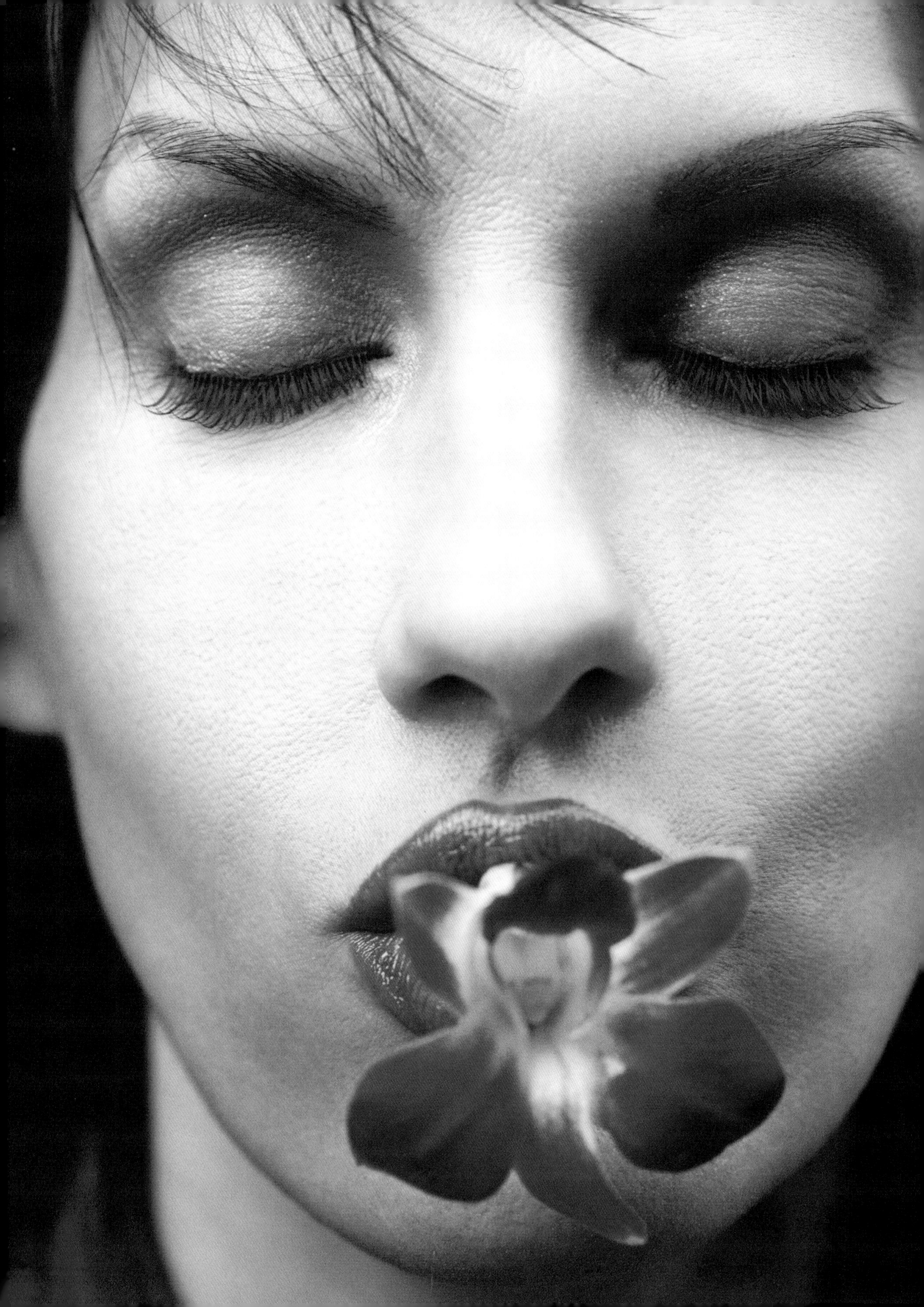

When I was in high school, I read about the beatnik poets and writers of the fifties and fantasized about moving to New York and becoming a writer in Greenwich Village. I related to the beat writers because they were not only subversive and artistic, but they were very sexual at a time when America was sexually repressed. So I moved to New York after college and began to write freelance articles for magazines and newspapers about various subjects, but always with a humor slant. It wasn't until I started writing for *Details*—a twenty-something men's "style" magazine—that I decided to write about sex, love, and dating. Hardly anybody was writing about sex at the time—and practically no women were. So after the third article, they offered me a column, which organically evolved from my own experiences. After writing the column for two years, I met Allen Ginsberg at a party and he asked me what I called myself. I told him I wasn't sure. "Sexual affairs correspondent" sounded like I was writing about someone's extramarital affairs. "Sexologist" wasn't quite right because I was writing about my own sex life—my sexual (mis)adventures in the first person. He told me to go with "sex columnist" since nobody else was calling themselves that. He told me to define what a sex columnist was. So I did.

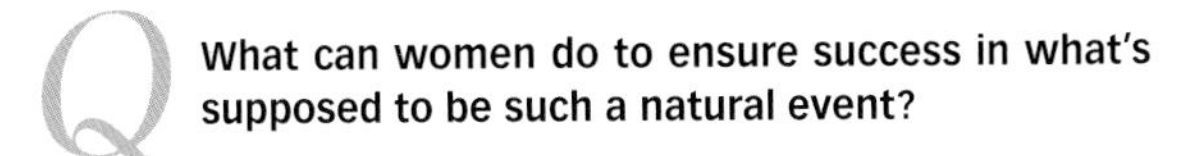

Q What can women do to ensure success in what's supposed to be such a natural event?

Sex is one of the most intimate and personal things we do with another person, yet we are embarrassed to talk about it with the person we are doing it with. I think people turn to "sex experts" because they want to have better sex. They want to enjoy it—which is good—but it's even more important to talk to the people they are having sex with. You have to ask for what you want. Sometimes women are dissatisfied with their sex lives and get mad at their boyfriends or husbands and just fume in silence. Then, if they reject their husbands or boyfriends sexually, the relationship gets worse. If a man is unhappy with his sexual relationship with a woman, he's probably unhappy with the relationship as a whole.

Q Instinct is a huge part of sensuality, yet women have such a hard time letting go of preconceived ideas about what looks sexy and instead going with their desires. How can we begin to relax and enjoy sex in such an image-conscious society?

Once you get into bed with someone, stop worrying about your fat thighs! Or your fat stomach, small boobs, or whatever body imperfection embarrasses you. By the time you're in bed, it's too late to worry about it. Don't compare yourself to fashion models, *Playboy* bunnies, or *Baywatch* babes. Relax and realize that the person who is in bed with you found you attractive enough to try to get you into bed in the first place. And once men are in bed with you, they are looking for things to turn them on, not off.

Q You must have answered thousands of questions from men during your years at *Details*. Could you give us some insight into the male sexual psyche?

Men are simple. Sex is very important to them. But even though they think about sex all the time, some men are still pretty bad at it. They want to please women sexually. They want women to enjoy sex as much as they do—not just lie there. But a lot of guys have no idea what women want. That's why we have to tell them what we like.

A lot of men ask how to perform oral sex. And—no surprise here—many men want to know how to last longer than two minutes! But the most ridiculous question I got lately was "How do I have sex with a woman without dating her?" In other words, "How can I have sex as quickly as possible without doing any work?"

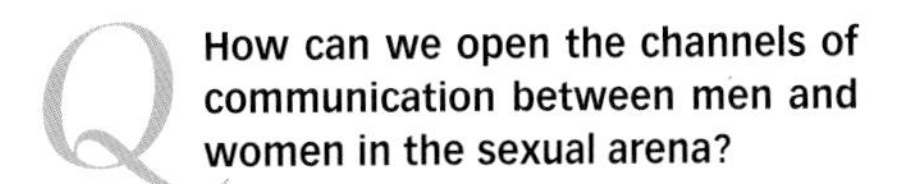

Q How can we open the channels of communication between men and women in the sexual arena?

I think sex is seen in a very negative light these days. People have grown afraid of sex as a result of the prevalence of sexually transmitted diseases, the frequent occurrences of sexual assault, and generally ignorant sexual behavior. But to truly enjoy sex, we have to overcome these negative experiences and fears and replace them with communication and information. We have to realize that sex is a pleasurable thing. Before we get into bed with our lover boy (toys) we have to mentally prepare ourselves for sex. "It's going to be fun," we have to think. I'm going to get excited and have an orgasm! And finally, *I* get to push *his* head down!

ANKA'S

Once you get into bed, **don't worry about how you look;** don't worry about what's too big or fat or small. Men want to get turned on, not turned off.

Don't put up with abuse or disrespectful behavior from men. Sometimes we let guys get away with not treating us well. If you start dating someone, and he says a couple of things that are demeaning or insulting, don't go out with him again. Those are red flags. When you first meet a man, he should be on his best behavior. If he makes you feel bad in any way, it's only going to get worse. The best relationships are based on mutual respect.

Ask for what you want in sex and in life. Men demand what they want all the time. Men are very direct. We need to tell men what we want. Be tactful and direct.

Sex is one of the most intimate and personal things we do with each other, but we don't talk to each other about it. **Tell men what you like in bed.** Then tell them what you don't like, too.

Relax, it's just sex. Don't get so nervous and uptight that you're not even enjoying it. Men don't want you to just lie there. Men enjoy sex and we should, too.

If you've experienced sexual abuse in your past, confront it. Talk about it with someone. Therapy can really help you move on. You have to let go of the anger toward the victimizer. It's over. If you don't confront and resolve it, you'll keep reliving it. Think of sex as something positive that makes you feel better, physically and emotionally.

Don't take anger or hurt from a past relationship into the next. Don't take it out on the person you are now with.

Take turns massaging each other. It will relax you before sex. And it's really sexy.

Courting and romance are part of the physiological warm-up to the physical act of sex. Today, courtship is somewhat lost. A lot of single guys want to get to the sex without the courtship. If a guy won't court you, you probably shouldn't have sex with him unless you just want a "sex buddy." If you do have a "sex buddy," don't get too emotional about him or you'll get hurt.

ADVICE

Women spend far more time talking about men than men do about women. While we're sitting around analyzing their psyches, men are analyzing our boobs. Men are simple. With that in mind, single women should adopt a more playgirl attitude toward men and just enjoy dating them.

You own your sexuality. And that is very powerful. Sex is a gift we give each other. Single and married women shouldn't have sex with their men unless they display respect and affection.

Mentally prepare yourself for sex. Men think about it all the time! Think of it as a pleasurable thing. Think, "I'm going to enjoy this. I'm going to get excited and have an orgasm." Sex is supposed to be fun.

If you are married and have kids, try to keep things fresh. Take a long weekend alone with your man or go on a fake honeymoon. Do it in a new position or weird place.

Never fake orgasms. He'll think you're satisfied and do even less work.

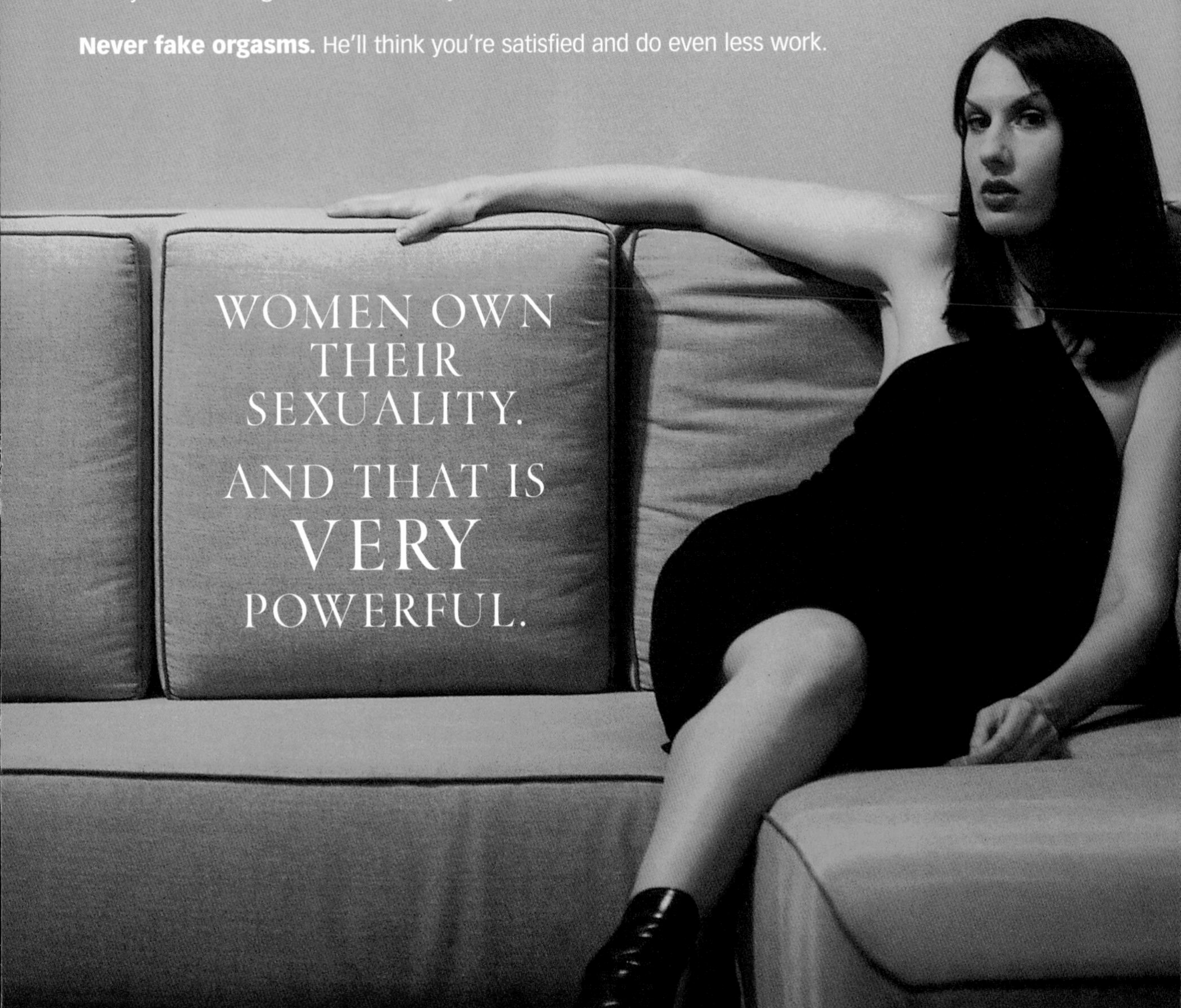

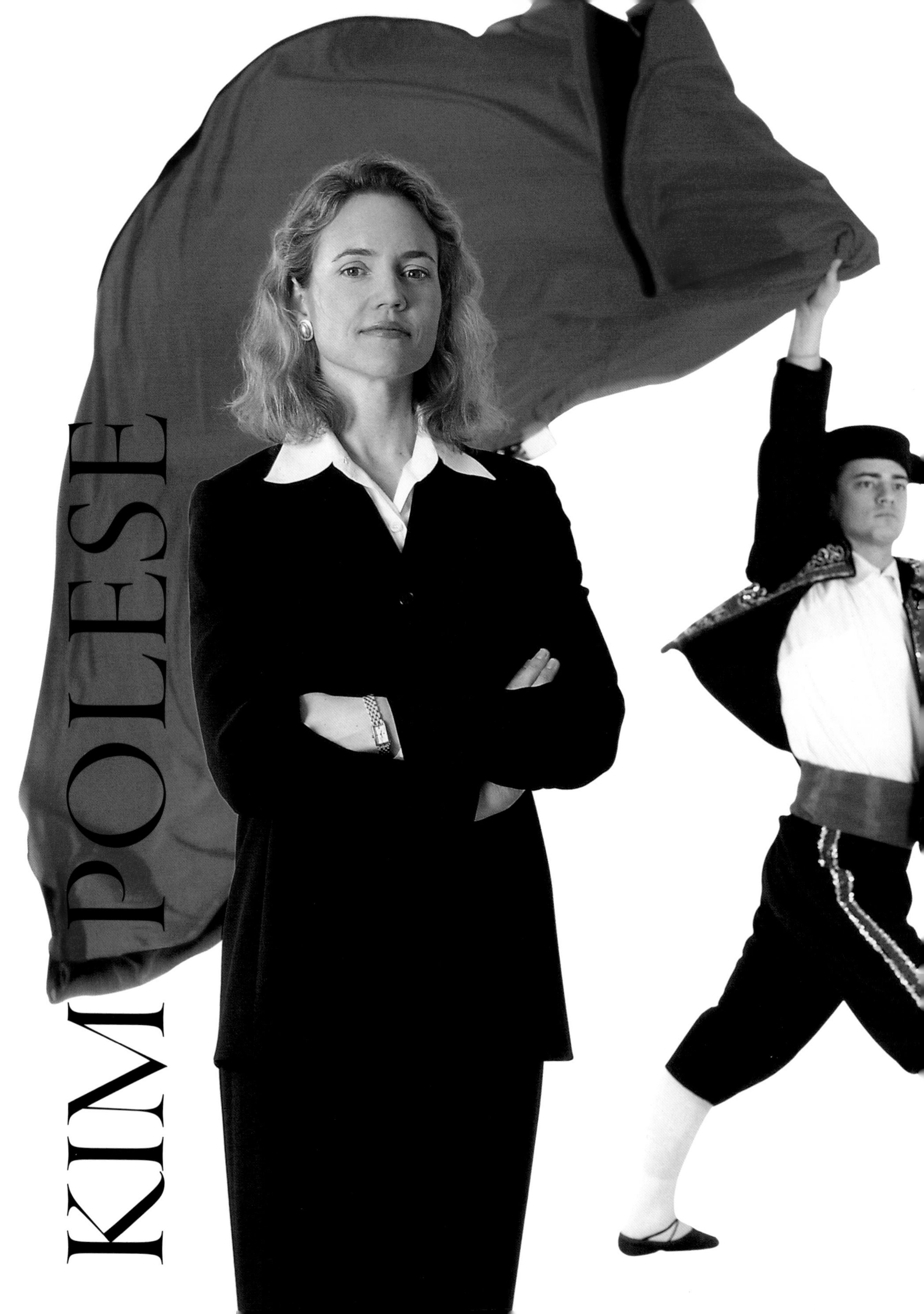
KIM POLESE

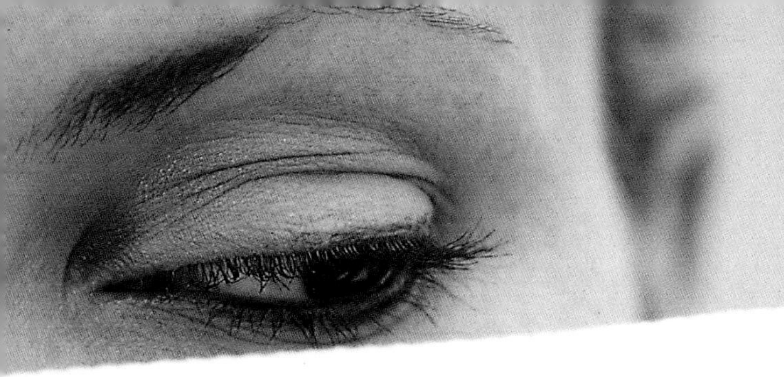

FOR STARTING A BUSINESS

Hire up. The caliber of the first people you hire is more important to the success or failure of your company than anything else. Hire better people than you think you need. And never hire friends over experience. People who are self-employed often fall into the trap of thinking that no one else can do the job as well as they will. Businesses based on fear are doomed to failure. A successful entrepreneur is someone who can achieve pre-determined goals through the efforts of herself and others.

Build value early. Build substance into your company before seeking start-up capital. Prepare a solid business plan, a prototype of your product (if applicable), and a compelling marketing/sales pitch before you approach investors. This will not only help with investors, it will also tell you where you are and give you the clarity to strategize about how you are going to get from point A to point B.

Get great legal advice up front. Find a good law firm to help with incorporation, navigating the world of venture capital, patent issues, and so on. Don't be afraid to give your valued advisors a little equity as incentive. These people will be critical in helping you get your company off the ground.

Go for smart money. When raising your initial capital, find an experienced investor who has backed other companies and been instrumental in helping them succeed. Make sure experience comes along with your start-up capital.

Don't focus on your "exit strategy." Plan on building your company for the long term, and everything else will follow. Remember, you don't just find what you're looking for, you create it.

Twenty-five years ago Sylvia Weinstock **was an elementary school teacher living on Long Island with her attorney husband and three daughters.** Many such women enjoy baking cakes but only one became the architect of America's confectionary dreams. After a diagnosis of breast cancer prompted a life change, Sylvia took up baking full time. "I always found food very nurturing," she says. Her client list now includes Donald Trump, Whitney Houston, Mariah Carey, Jane Fonda, Hillary Clinton, Oprah Winfrey, and everyone who's anyone. But according to her clients, whether ordering a cake for twenty or two thousand, anyone who walks into Sylvia's shop is treated like royalty.

SYLVIA WEINSTOCK

Q Sylvia, you requested that I photograph you with your three great friends. Tell me about these women you so admire.

Between the four of us, we range in age from sixty-five to eighty-five. These three women are super achievers as well as great friends.

Judith Leiber's Hungarian Jewish family barely escaped the Nazis. Many relatives were not so lucky. The handiwork of a neighbor who forged a visa for her family is the reason she is here today.

Judith singlehandedly put handbags on the map. Many women consider it a rite of passage for a woman to get a Judith Leiber handbag when she turns forty or fifty. It means that she has arrived. Leiber handbags are on display all over the world, including the Met. Each bag contains up to ten thousand Austrian rhinestones applied by hand. Among the women who carry and collect them are Elizabeth Taylor, Barbara Walters, and Queen Elizabeth. All of her clients proclaim her as the last of the greats.

Judith loves to bring other women joy through her work. I think a person's humanity and love for people translates into a love of her work and Judith creates a product that reflects her dignity.

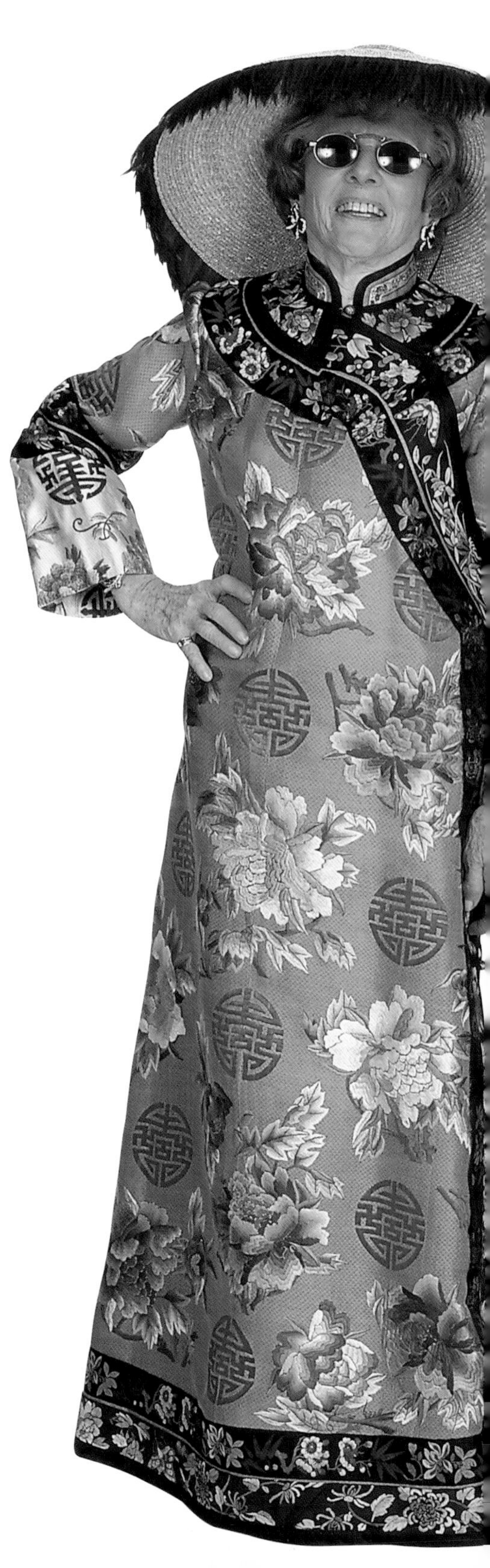

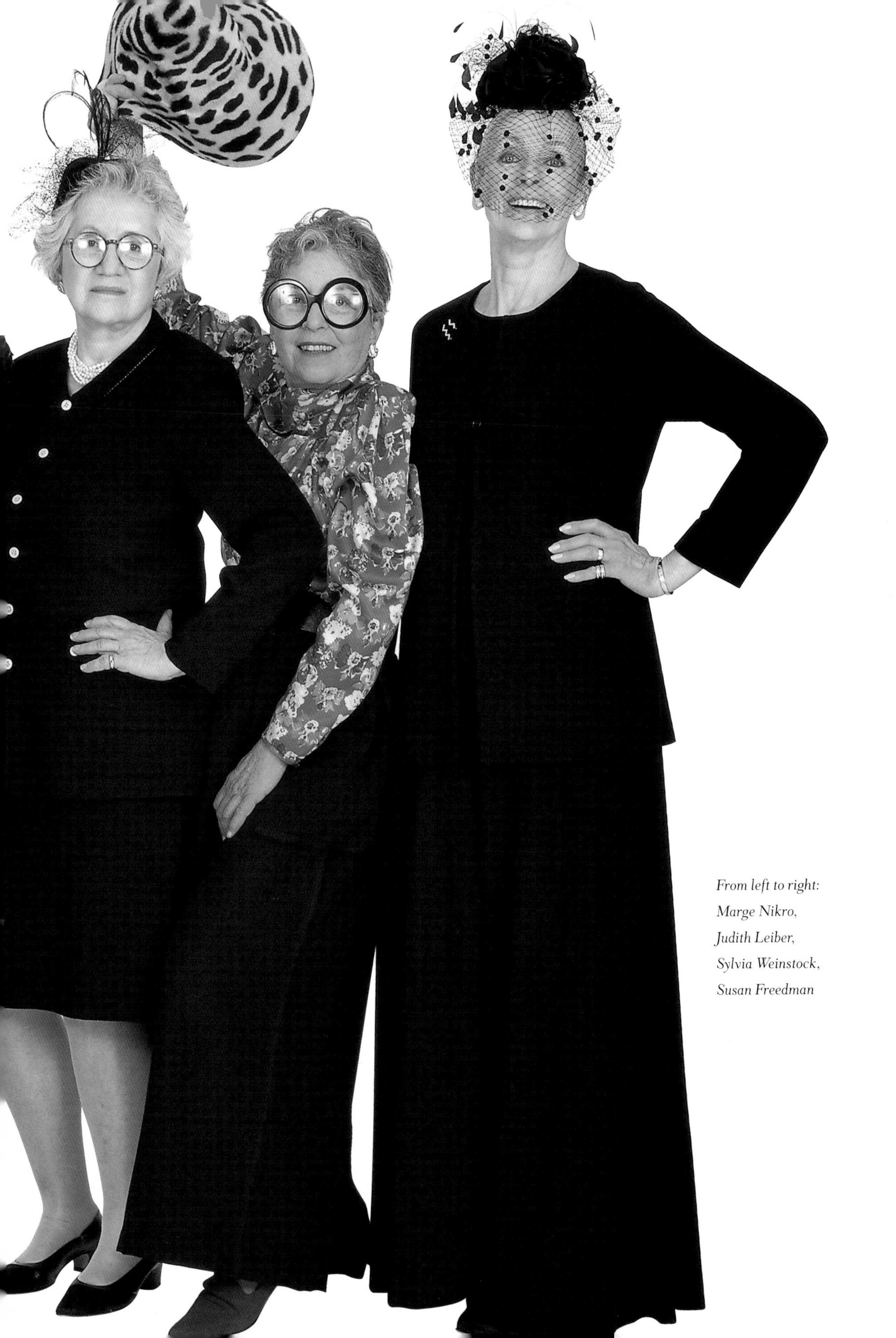

From left to right: Marge Nikro, Judith Leiber, Sylvia Weinstock, Susan Freedman

Marge Nikro was a trailblazer in the photography world. She was the first to exhibit erotic photography as an art form. She was also the first person the Hell's Angels allowed to exhibit photographs taken of them—she even invited them to tea.

Her mother died of breast cancer when she was a little girl. Her father and brothers raised her to be uninhibited and independent, which helped her through her own bout with breast cancer. It also led her to start several businesses, the most infamous being the Nikro Gallery, which she opened almost thirty years ago. She was the first person to show Robert Maplethorpe's work. She also had a monthly show called *Rated X*, which displayed erotica as art. They lined up around the block for that one!

But Marge was more than a gallery owner. She was also a mentor to many young photographers. She never let an artist show her a portfolio without trying to inspire them. No matter how bad the work was, no one left her gallery feeling like giving up. This, she feels, is the key to longevity—taking all of your knowledge and spreading it around. Be inspiring and your wisdom will carry on.

Susan Freedman works in fabric development for Clarence House, which is considered the finest decorative fabrics house in the industry. She has been a mentor to many young designers and has helped to implement the design of famous institutions all over the world.

She started thirty years ago in the interior design marketing and public relations business. In those days working women were still scarce. But Susan loved to work. And today she thinks that as women age, they need to stay active in body, mind, and spirit, and to not give in to society's standards of youth. They just have to keep going. She tells her younger colleagues, "When the door closes, a window will open. There is always another avenue to take. When an opportunity comes along, take it. The worst thing that can happen is that you take another road in the long run."

Q **I understand that being diagnosed with breast cancer twenty years ago was the impetus behind your baking career. That must have had a huge impact on your outlook on life.**

I found that cancer myself. I went to the doctor, and he couldn't find it because it was smaller than a pea. It didn't even show up on any mammography tests. But I was not satisfied, so I asked my doctor to take it out. When he did that, he found that it was indeed cancerous. I was lucky I didn't wait because it had already started to spread. It was quite a scare but I never had any doubt that I was going to be fine in the end. In fact, my doctor took me on as a patient because he so liked my attitude. One night, while recovering in the hospital after my mastectomy, I snuck out to attend a function with my husband, tucking the drain tube running from my armpit into my jacket pocket. Although I returned in just two short hours my oncologist caught me. I was terrified that he would drop me as a patient, but instead he told me that I was a winner because it was obvious that nothing was going to stop me. To this day the oncologist calls to ask me to do telephone hand-holding with some of his more frightened patients. I tell them that cancer had a very positive affect on me—it gave me a great sense of value. I began to realize that I can do anything I want to do. And now something that would have upset me before I had cancer no longer upsets me. If something doesn't happen the way I want it to, I say to myself, "Well, it's not cancer." I have gained a great sense of perspective.

It was while I was undergoing chemotherapy that I started my bakery business. My husband, Ben, was distressed at the idea of me traveling back and forth from the city for treatment. So he decided to give up his law practice, and just like that we sold everything and moved to New York. He became my driving force, as well as my delivery boy. Baking had always been such a passion of mine. It was so enveloping that I had no time to be tired or feel ill. It was a fantastic way to focus my energy on life instead of cancer.

Q **You have a zest for life and learning. I know that you have quite a collection of degrees. What is it about the bakery business that feeds that passion?**

I see life as a bag of tricks. You have in that bag all your skills and knowledge—it makes you who you are and you can always be changing and growing but only if you are open to learning from others. My business allows me to

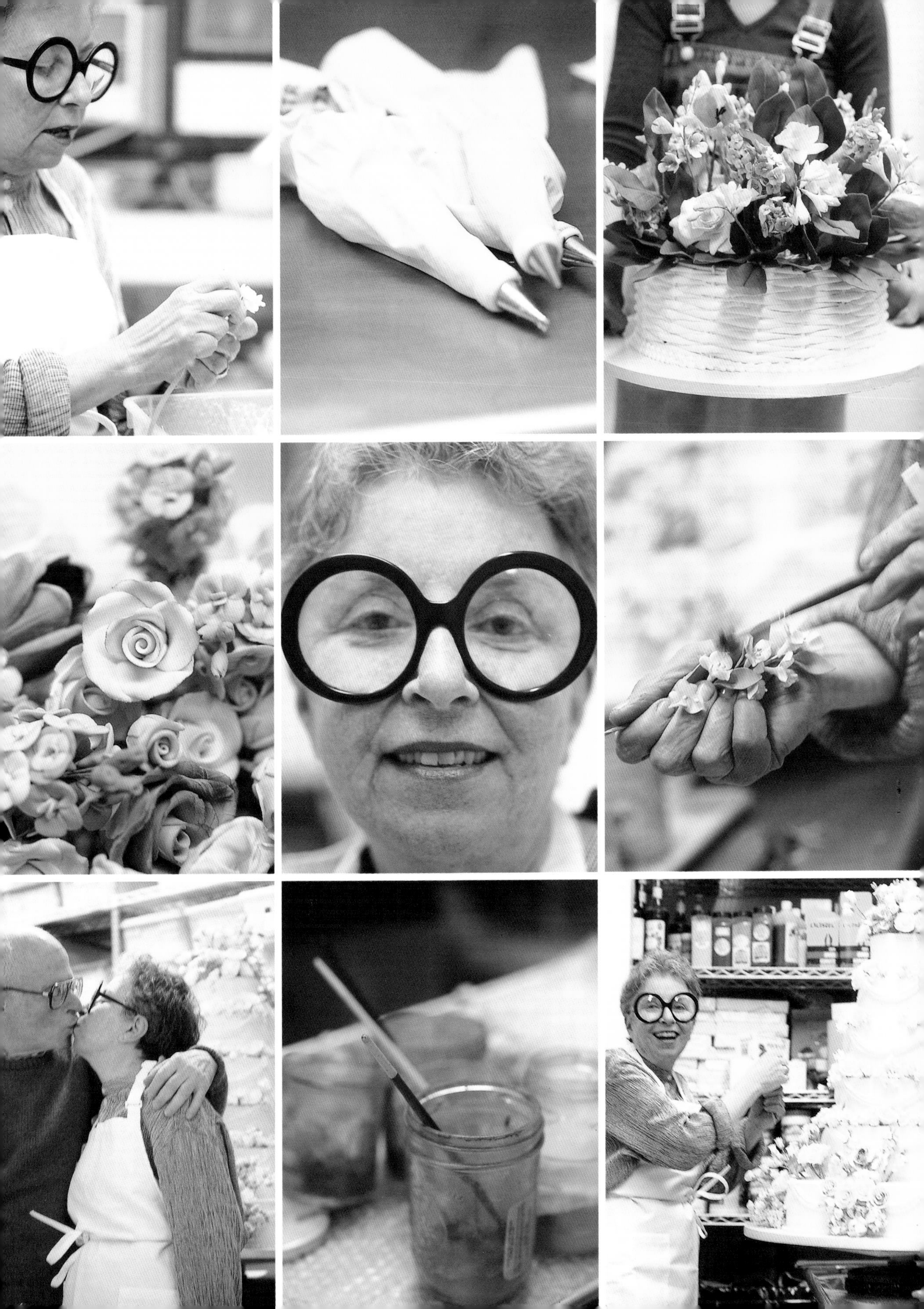

constantly expand my bag of tricks. It also enabled me to meet so many people who have enriched my life—from housewives and schoolteachers to socialites and celebrities. Yesterday I met with an aunt, a mother, and the bride—all of whom were schoolteachers—and we discussed how to improve the school system. The other day I had someone from Wall Street here, and we talked about the internet and stocks. Then I saw a professor who is part of the agricultural department at one of the local universities and we talked about genetically engineered foods.

People and learning have always fascinated me. That's why I earned degrees in psychology, education psychology, and a bachelor's in education. I apply that knowledge in my business every day. You practically have to be a psychiatrist to know how to please your client. People want events to be memorable and meaningful. They want to express themselves. You have to be able to assess their needs because they often don't know what they want and are coming to you for advice.

Q In your business you work closely with a lot of wedding parties. You also have a successful marriage yourself. You must have a lot of insight into the whole process and institution of marriage.

Many women develop a kind of Hollywood illusion of love. They want to be courted and have a fairy-tale wedding. But very often they don't even know what love is all about. A lot of couples are unprepared for the realities of marriage, like having the same person in bed next to you every morning, dealing with illness, sharing chores, and coping with dual finances. They haven't even discussed the most simple aspects of sharing a life. It takes a lot of ingredients to make a marriage work—love, nurturing, compromise, respect, chemistry, common interests, giving each other space. And the most important thing for yourself and your marriage is not sweating the small stuff. Let it go. Look upon an argument and say, "What if one of us drops dead this second? Is this argument that important? What does it really mean in the summation of a lifetime?"

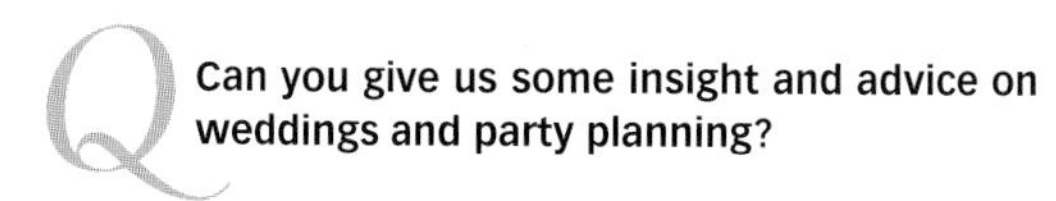

Q Can you give us some insight and advice on weddings and party planning?

A lot of weddings have lost their meaning today. Everyone wants bigger and grander. People stretch their financial limits too far when they should do the best they can within their price range. I love to see people reaching for less quantity and more quality. Otherwise, the wedding becomes a high-pressure event that has to be perfect and loses its essence. Women obsess over the exact color of the ribbon or the size of the invitations. It is not unusual for me to get late-night phone calls six months before the wedding from a panicking bride who can't sleep before she lets me know that she's changed her colors from pink to peach. She's certain to never enjoy her wedding.

There is also the all-too-common problem of the power struggle between daughter and mother. Mothers want to mother and daughters want to assert their independence. It's nice to see mothers giving guidance but usually it just ends up in a big fight. And for what? Again, the whole spirit of the event vanishes. I say, keep it simple, stay within your financial means, don't sweat each and every detail, and enjoy yourself. I frequently ask, "Who's going to remember this twenty years down the line?" No one is going to notice if the pink of the flowers is the exact same pink as the bridesmaids' dresses. What they will remember is the happiness you give people and your own sense of integrity. Was your day filled with love and sharing? Honesty, integrity, loyalty toward friends, and openness to accepting new ideas—these are the important parts of life to focus on. When you bring that sort of an attitude to the planning of the wedding, it will always be wonderful.

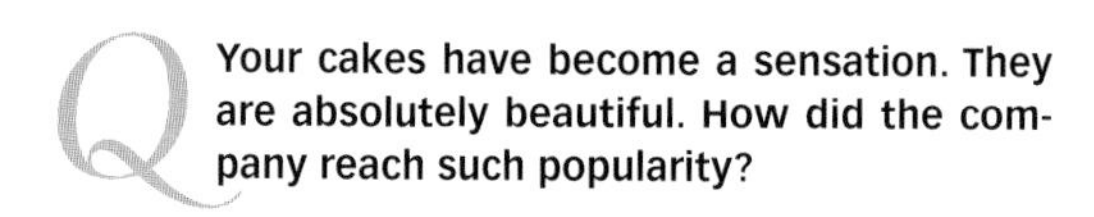

Q Your cakes have become a sensation. They are absolutely beautiful. How did the company reach such popularity?

Very early on, someone wanted a cake for a wedding, so my husband and I drove it to the wedding caterer's shop. The caterer was so impressed with the cake that he put it in his window, where it was seen by a chef who worked for Daniel Bruce White, one of the best caterers in New York. They became one of my customers and through them we got some of the best parties in town. High-society ladies started ordering our cakes and we started to get top billing. We were the new kids in town and the first to make a cake that is

“YOU CAN NEVER
RE-CREATE THE PAST—
BUT YOU CAN SHAPE
YOUR OWN FUTURE
AND YOU CAN
MAKE A CAKE.”

—JACQUELINE DEVAL

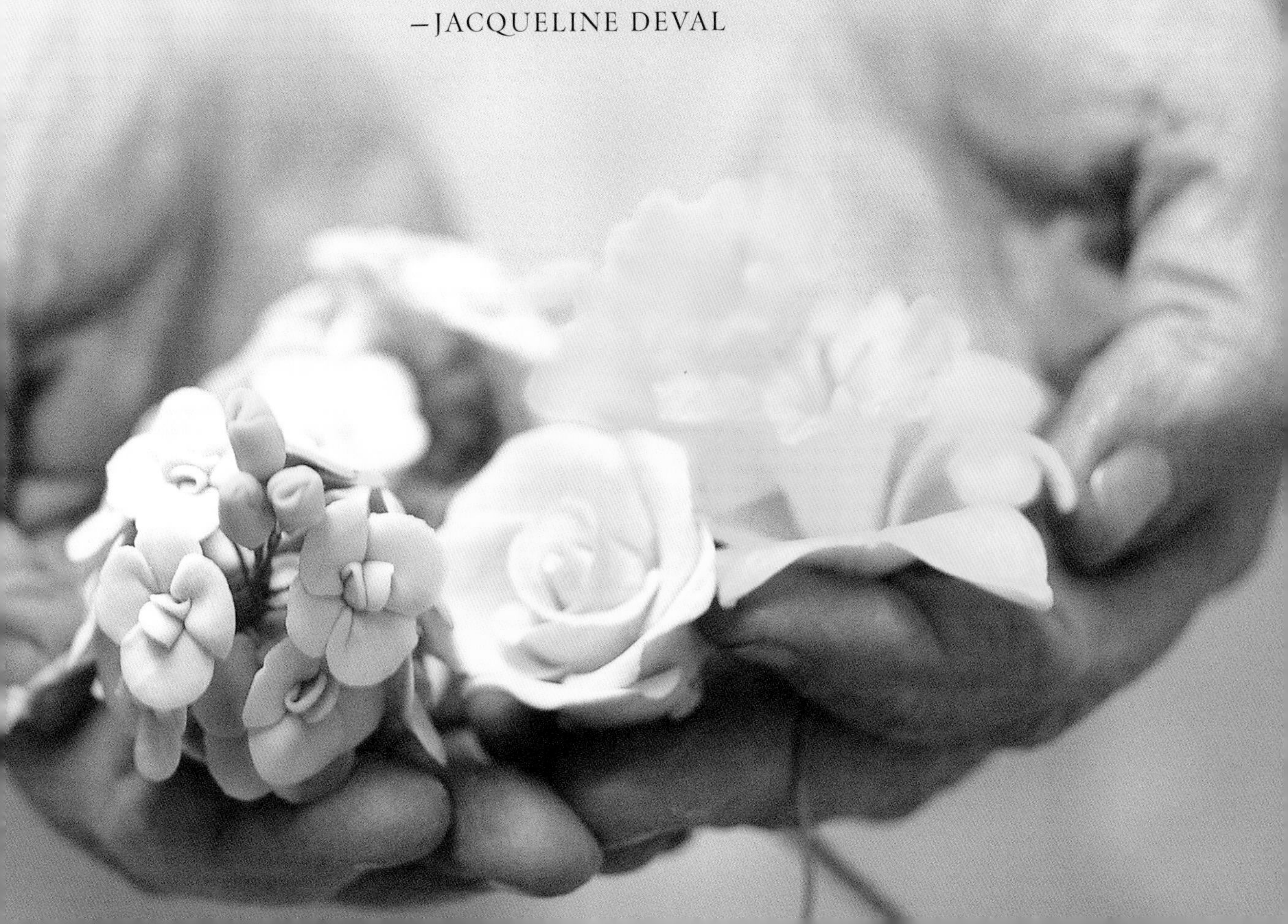

beautiful and also delicious. The funny part of this story is that the initial cake that went into the caterer's window had been in an accident on the way over in the car. We had stopped short and the cake had gotten smashed. I sent Ben back to the shop to get more flowers and we just loaded that cake with flowers to cover the disaster. I guess it worked.

Q You transport enormous cakes to events all over the world. Do you have any standout stories about getting cakes to faraway places?

There is always the challenge of flying with the cakes. They are always chaperoned by me or one of my employees, and we always carry extra flowers and icing, just in case. There are also special considerations depending on which country you are delivering to. For example, when we send cakes to Saudi Arabia, I only send male employees. And there is the all-important detail of whether or not the cake will fit through the door of the plane. We have had that problem before. Sometimes we can't take the cakes ourselves because of international customs, so we have to help the client pack it and give them instructions on how to assemble it when they arrive. In one situation there were ten members of a family traveling by air, and each one took a section of the cake in their carry-on luggage.

Q You talk a lot about how, for women, baking is a cathartic experience. You've even called it erotic. Give me your spin on the relationship between food and pleasure.

Baking is a tactile thing. It's a wonderful feeling to mix with your hands, blend your egg whites, and feel the silkiness of the batter running between your fingers. Even flower-making is tactile—you know when your petal is too thick because you can feel it in your hand. Working with the dough is a sensual feeling. It's like silk or satin. I feel like a baby who sucks the edge of a blanket. In today's world women are overwhelmed by the busyness of life and conflicting emotions, they need a chance to stop and smell the roses (or bake them). There is a great saying by Jacqueline Deval, "You can never re-create the past. But you can shape your own future. And you can make a cake."

Sylvia Weinstock's Classic Yellow Cake

2 1/4 cups sifted cake flour
2 teaspoons baking powder
1/2 teaspoon salt
1/2 pound (two sticks) unsalted butter, at room temperature
2 cups sugar
2 large egg yolks
2 teaspoons vanilla
4 large egg whites
1 cup sour cream

Preheat oven to 350 degrees. Butter two 8-by-8 inch baking pans and line with parchment.

Sift together the flour, baking powder, and salt. Set aside.

Cream the butter in a large bowl with an electric mixer until fluffy and light in color, about 2 minutes on medium speed. Add the sugar and continue to mix until fluffy and light.

Then add the egg yolks, one at a time, making sure each is thoroughly incorporated before adding the next one. Add the vanilla.

Reduce the mixer speed to low and add the dry ingredients alternately with the sour cream, beginning and ending with the flour. Be sure the mixture is completely blended after each addition. Scrape the sides of the bowl, and beat for 1 minute longer.

In a separate bowl, with clean beaters, beat the egg whites to soft peaks. Gently fold the whipped whites into the batter with a rubber spatula.

Pour the batter into the prepared pans and smooth the tops with a rubber spatula. Bake 45 to 50 minutes. The top of the cake should be nicely browned. Test for doneness with a toothpick. Insert it into the center and it should come out dry and clean.

Basic Buttercream Icing

1 1/4 cups sugar
1 pound (4 sticks) unsalted butter, at room temperature, cut into 1/2 sticks
4 large egg whites
2 tablespoons clear vanilla extract
1/4 cup water

In a medium saucepan, combine the sugar and water, mixing with a wooden spoon until the sugar is dissolved. Place the pan on the stove and use a clean pastry brush to paint the area just above the water line with water. Turn the burner to medium and heat, watching the sugar mixture to be sure it does not caramelize or burn. Put a candy thermometer in the pan and simmer the sugar-water mixture without stirring, until the thermometer reaches 240 degrees (soft-ball stage); this will take about 5 to 7 minutes.

As the sugar nears the required temperature, place the egg whites in the large bowl of an electric mixer. Using a wire whisk attachment, beat the egg whites at medium speed until they begin to hold soft peaks (3 to 5 minutes) and double in volume. Do not overbeat.

Turn the mixer on high and very carefully and slowly pour the hot sugar mixture in a very thin stream near the edge of the bowl and into the beaten egg whites. Beat for 20 to 35 minutes on medium to high speed. The egg whites will lose some of their volume and the mixture should resemble a very thick meringue. The outside of the bowl should be slightly warm to the touch.

At this point, reduce the speed to medium or low and add the room-temperature butter pieces, one at a time. The mixture will break and begin to look like cottage cheese, but don't worry. Keep the mixer running, continue adding butter, and let the mixer whip the buttercream until it begins to get smooth again; this could take up to 10 minutes. Once the mixture is smooth, add the vanilla and beat for 5 minutes more. The buttercream is now ready to be colored or chilled. (If the buttercream is too soft, chill for 10 minutes and then beat again. If this doesn't work, cream 1 tablespoon of chilled butter, and then gently add the creamed butter to the buttercream. Beat until smooth and without lumps.)

Yield: 4 cups

Basic Buttercream Filling

5 egg yolks
2 cups sugar
$^1/_3$ cup water
1 egg
$1^1/_2$ pounds (6 sticks) unsalted butter at room temperature, cut into $^1/_2$ sticks
6 tablespoons vanilla extract or $^1/_3$ to $^1/_2$ cup flavored liqueur

Place the egg yolks in the large bowl of an electric mixer. Using a wire whisk attachment, beat at medium speed until the mixture turns from orange to pale yellow. Continue whisking while you proceed with the next step.

In a medium saucepan, combine the sugar and $^1/_3$ cup water with a wooden spoon until the sugar is dissolved. Place the pan on the stove and use a clean pastry brush to paint the area just above the water line with water. Turn the heat to medium and heat, watching the sugar mixture to be sure that it doesn't caramelize or burn. Put a candy thermometer in the pan and simmer until the thermometer reaches 240 degrees (soft-ball stage); this will take 5 to 7 minutes.

With the mixer still running on medium speed, very carefully and slowly pour the hot sugar mixture in a very thin stream down the side of the bowl (near the edge) and into the yolks. (Do not pour the hot sugar all at once directly into the middle of the eggs.) Beat for 12 to 15 minutes on medium speed, or until the outside of the bowl is slightly warm to the touch.

Add the butter pieces, one at a time. The mixture may break and begin to look like cottage cheese, but don't worry. Keep the mixer running and continue adding butter. Beat until it begins to get smooth again. This could take up to 10 minutes. Once the mixture is smooth, add the vanilla or other flavoring and beat for 3 minutes more. (If the filling is too soft, chill for 10 minutes before you fill the cake. If the filling is still soft, cream 4 tablespoons chilled butter and then gently whip the creamed butter into the filling, 1 tablespoon at a time.) The filling may be stored in an airtight container in the refrigerator for up to 5 days.

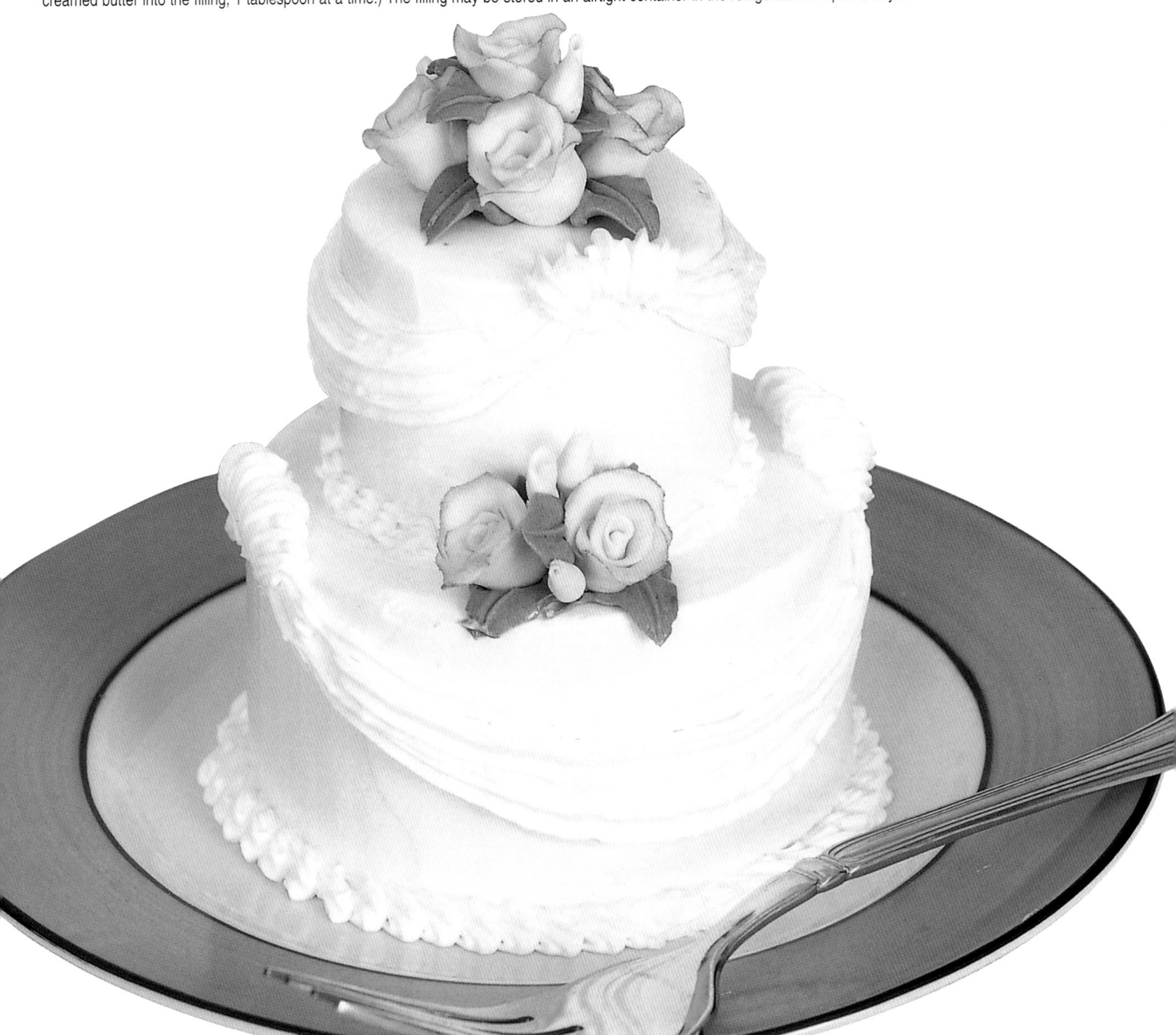

Tea Without

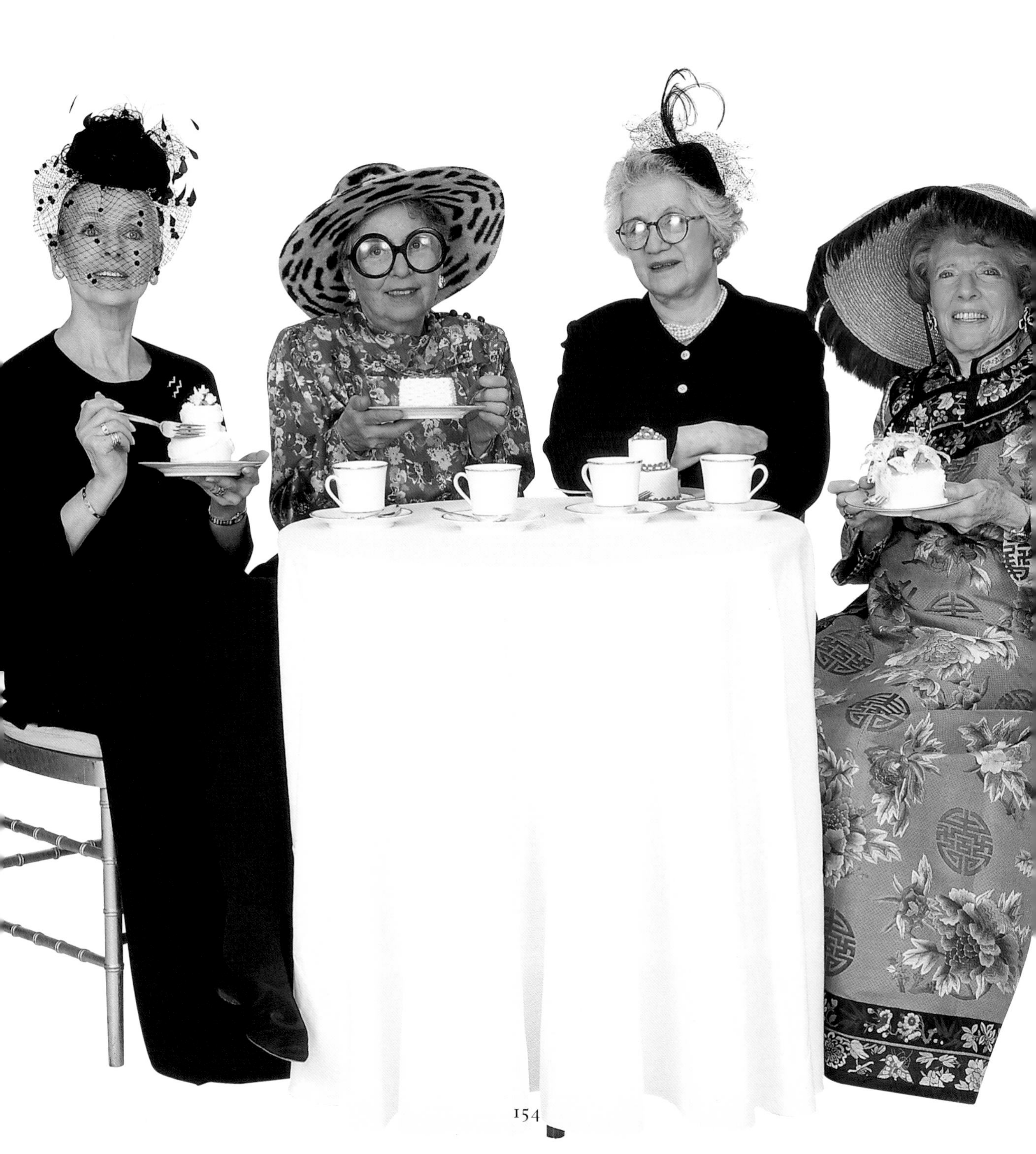

Sympathy

Life Lessons from Ladies Who've Lived and Learned

Seek the advice of others, but never give over too much authority too soon.

Have a clear concept of what you want to accomplish in life. Ask yourself: What am I planning to get out of this? Will I have integrity? Will I be honest with myself?

Keep an even keel. Being a person of even keel means that you don't get thrown by catastrophes. All of the most successful people have been able to let go of disaster very quickly and move on.

Work hard. People don't seem to work as hard today. They want immediate gratification, but instead they should think of the long term. In our day we didn't think about benefits when we first started out—we were willing to work for nothing in order to learn a trade and become accomplished. People need to realize that life lasts a lot longer than you think and what you do today can profoundly affect your future.

Believe in your product. In business, whatever you do you will have competition. And never copy an existing product—you will always be a step behind a more established business and anxious to catch up. Make sure your product has integrity. Luck will find you if you get the right product out there.

Try new things. As women age, they are not encouraged to branch out and do new things. We work with women in their nineties who are creating new and amazing art all the time.

Be honest. When you deal with yourself with a sense of honesty, you deal with other people in the same way.

Be brave. You have to learn to be very brave to follow a dream. It's also important to be cautious and diligent, but if you feel something in your heart, you need to be brave and just do it. You never know if something is going to work, but the worst thing that can happen is you fail. Failure is rarely fatal.

Cultivate friendship. It is a critical part of a fulfilled life.

Marriage is the same as business; you have to work through the good times and the bad times without panicking. Decide if your relationship is worthy. Do you love your partner? Rather than focusing on whether or not you like the way he puts his clothes away, think about how he treats you. All four of us had good men behind us who encouraged our work. It has to be give and take.

Be a mentor. Women with wisdom need to share it with the younger generations but also teach them to think for themselves, to be dependent on themselves. You have to run your own lives. Remember, in the final analysis, it's your life.

Like yourself. You have to like what you're doing, whether it's going to work or raising children. You have to be challenged; each day your life must give you a purpose. Don't be a negative person; find the joy in all things possible.

Like what you do. There are a lot of things that we have to do that don't bring us instant pleasure but in the long run will give us satisfaction. Too many young people today say they don't like this or that. They have to put instant pleasure aside and work hard on all aspects of their lives—mental growth as well as intellectual growth. By putting some pleasures aside in the beginning, success will come in the long run. It can come in many forms: a business that brings monetary rewards, a loving relationship, rearing children who are capable and decent.

RESOURCES

For more information about the women in this book, please consult the following:

Sarah Ban Breathnach

Ban Breathnach, Sarah. *Simple Abundance: A Daybook of Comfort and Joy.* New York: Warner Books, 1995.

www.simpleabundance.com

Bobbi Brown

Brown, Bobbi, and Annemarie Iverson. *Bobbi Brown Beauty: The Ultimate Beauty Resource.* New York: HarperCollins, 1997.

www.bobbibrowncosmetics.com

Carolyn Dean

Dean, Carolyn, M.D. *Carolyn Dean's Complementary Natural Prescriptions for Common Ailments.* New Canaan, Conn.: Keats Publishing, 1994.

holeopharm@polnet.com

Sharon Gannon

The Jivamukti Yoga Center
404 Lafayette Street, 3rd Floor
New York, NY 10003 (212) 353-0214

www.jivamuktiyoga.com

Abby Hitchcock

Camaje Restaurant
85 Macdougal Street
New York, NY 10012 (212) 673-8184

Donna Karan

Sischy, Ingrid. *Donna Karan New York.* New York: Universe Publishing, 1998.

www.donnakaran.com

Nina Kelly

Soho Health Arts
470 Broome Street
New York, NY 10012 (212) 226-7551

Marcia Kilgore

Bliss Spas
www.blissworld.com

Judith Leiber

Judith Leiber Bags
20 West 33rd Street
New York, NY 10001 (212) 736-4244

Ellen McGirt

www.cassandrasrevenge.com

Verna Moses

Ultra Marathon Cycling
One Olympic Plaza
Colorado Springs, CO 80909 (719) 578-4581

Christiane Northrup

P. O. Box 199
Yarmouth, ME 04096
www.drnorthrup.com

Northrup, Christiane, M.D. *Women's Bodies, Women's Wisdom: Creating Physical and Emotional Health and Healing.* New York: Bantam Books, 1998.

Kim Polese

www.marimba.com

Anka Radakovich

Radakovich, Anka. *The Wild Girls Club: Tales from Below the Belt.* New York: Fawcett Books, 1995.

lalagel@aol.com

Cynthia Rowley

550 Seventh Avenue
New York, NY 10018 (212) 575-9020

Rowley, Cynthia, and Ilene Rosenzweig. *Swell: A Girl's Guide to the Good Life.* New York: Warner Books, 1999.

Kathy Smith

www.kathysmithlifestyles.com
www.womenssportsfoundation.org

Trudy Styler

The Rainforest Foundation
270 Lafayette Street, Suite 7
New York, NY 10012 (212) 431-9098

Taylor, Martha. *Eight Strategies For More Effective Giving,* The Women's Philanthropy Institute website (www.Women-philanthropy.org), 2000.

www.savetherest.org

Iyanla Vanzant

Inner Visions Worldwide Network
926 Philadelphia Avenue
Silver Springs, MD 20910 (301) 608-8750

Vanzant, Iyanla. *In the Meantime: Finding Yourself and the Love You Want.* New York: Simon & Schuster, 1999.

Vanzant, Iyanla. *One Day My Soul Just Opened Up: 40 Days and 40 Nights Towards Spiritual Strength and Personal Growth.* New York: Simon & Schuster, 1998.

www.innervisionsworldwide.com

Sylvia Weinstock

Sylvia Weinstock Cakes, Ltd.
273 Church Street
New York, NY 10013 (212) 925-6698

SINCERE THANKS

Thank you God for allowing me to live healthfully and do what I love the most, and for continuing to surround me with angels.

Thank you to all of the brilliant women who were so giving of their time and energy in order to be included in this book, especially Sharon Gannon for her generous assistance, words of encouragement, inspiring ideas, and friendship. Behind each of these great women was another great woman without whose invaluable help this book would not have been possible: Kristin Lee at Jivamukti Yoga, Jocelyn at Simple Abundance, Beth Mann at Bobbi Brown, Bernadette at Inner Visions, Suzan Woods at Marimba, Patti Cohen at Donna Karan, Celeste and Lauren at Cynthia Rowley, Mara Stern at Bliss, Erica at Kathy Smith, Ann and Theresa with Trudy Styler, Diane Grover with Dr. Christiane Northrup, Annie at Morgane Le Fay, Debra at Sony, and Dana at Lola Hats. Much gratitude to Rick Schwab and Beth Phillips for all of their help. Thank you to Patty Sicular at Ford Models for the great references; to Wendy and Oscar at the Oscar Bond Salon for the quick change; to everyone at the Joseph Ciccone Salon for helping with makeover madness; to all of the talented makeup artists, Dana, Julie, and Orlando–you made everyone even more beautiful. Thanks to Mr. Lenny at Something Special for all the bagels and faxes; Cherie for listening and writing without any complaints; Julie and Amanda at the Puck Building for all of their enthusiasm and the great work space; Liana Fredley for her skillful proofreading; and everyone at Flower Films, especially Chris Miller. Thanks, Dad, for everything. Thank you Heidi Volpe for getting the ball rolling and being a great friend. Thanks D–as usual, you saved the day with your creative genius and unbending work ethic. Thank you Kathy Nastase for all of your kindnesses toward Jake and for always greeting me with a smile. Thanks to my sister Francesca, who gave my son unending hours of love, and to Charles Miers, Bonnie Eldon, Belinda Hellinger, and Alex Tart at Universe for turning my dream into a reality, yet again.

For my husband, Owen, and my son, Jake, the love that I have for both of you is indescribable. The love I get from you is endless. Thank you.

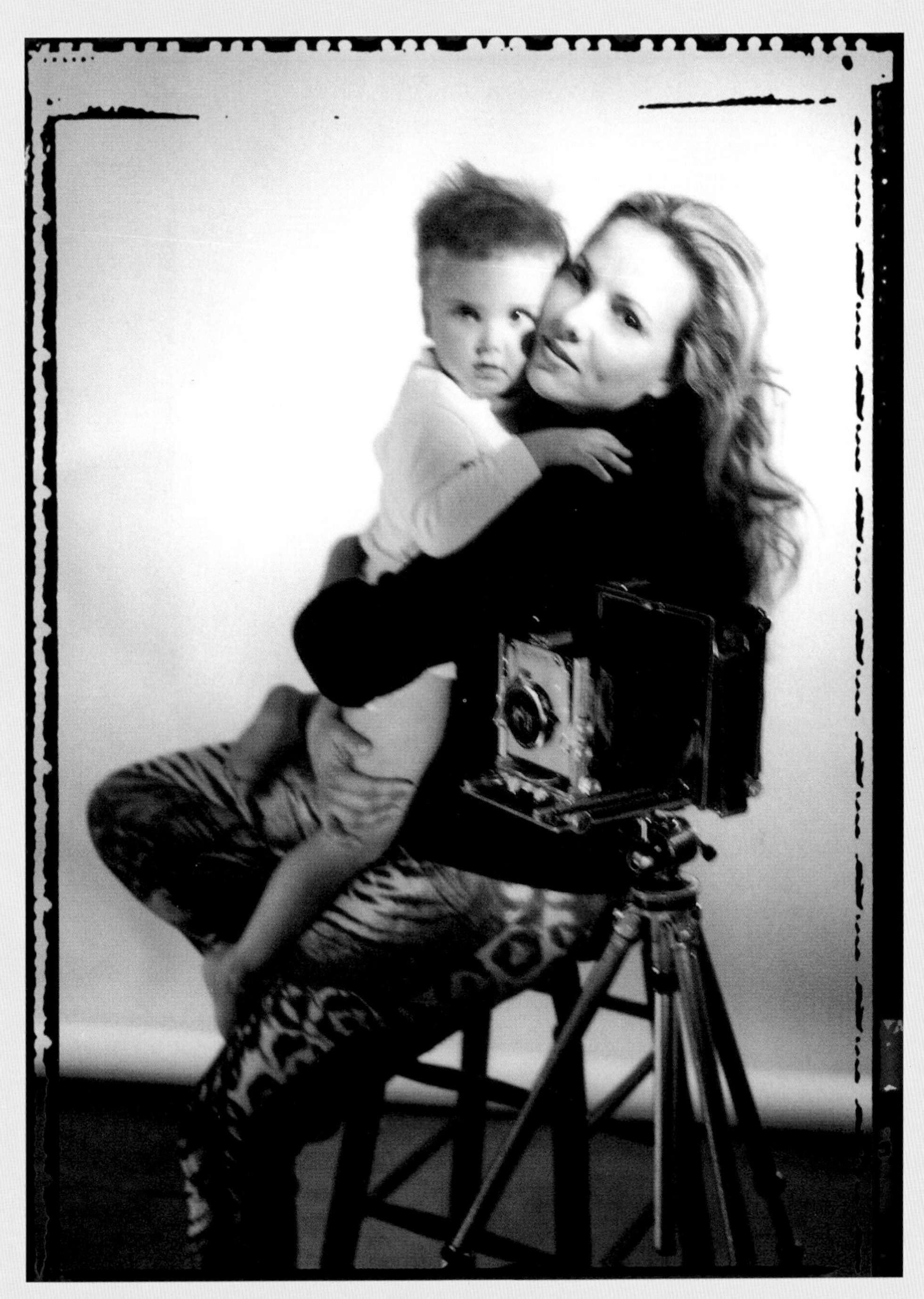

Christina Lessa and son Jake, New York, 2000

CREDITS

Associate editor: Cherie Turner. Hats provided by: Lola Hats, NYC. Wardrobe provided by: Morgane Le Fay.

Additional photos provided by: Ken Schles, Inc. (page 127); © Marc Baptiste/Outline (pages 20–21 and 23); © Peggy Sirota/Outline (pages 24–25); Cory Berrinson (page 106); Mikeal Jannson (pages 62–63).

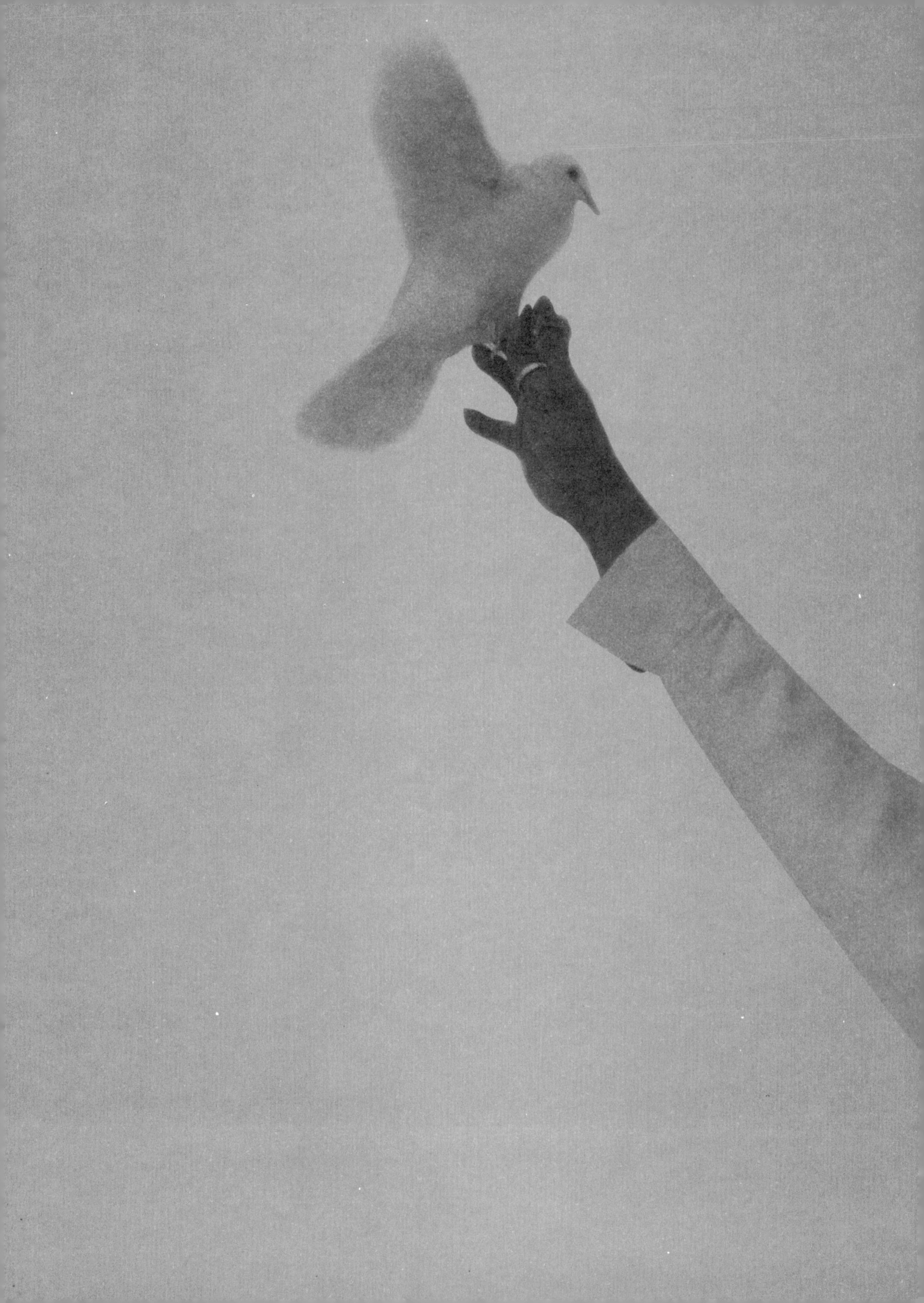